7 HEALTHY GUT HABITS FOR WOMEN OVER 40

GET YOUR LIFE BACK USING INTERMITTENT FASTING, NUTRITION, AND SELF-CARE TO RESTORE GUT MICROBIOME FOR WEIGHT LOSS AND INCREASED ENERGY

LARA WEST

CONTENTS

YOUR GIFT

7 HEALTHY GUT HABITS FOR WOMEN OVER 40 WORKBOOK

The habits described in this book are simple and easy to follow. Once you form them, you'll be well on your way to a healthier, more fulfilling life, to a lifestyle you love, and to making your 40s and beyond your best years.

However, it's often difficult to make consistent positive changes and stick to new habits.

I created this workbook to help you succeed. You can track your habits in multiple ways in different worksheets. It's important to be conscious of your thoughts and committed to your new habits, and take small steps. Record your intentions, plans, thoughts, and results in the workbook. Strive for progress, not perfection. Forgive yourself when you skip a day. Commit to the next action. Reward yourself for every check-mark on your list. Give your best to form the habits, and before you know it, your new habits will give you your life back.

Get immediate access to the bonus by following this link https://larawestbooks.com/workbook or scanning this QR Code:

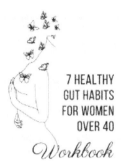

INTRODUCTION

> *Quite literally, your gut is the epicenter of your mental and physical health. If you want better immunity, efficient digestion, improved clarity, and balance, focus on rebuilding your gut health.*
>
> — KRIS CARR, NEW YORK TIMES BEST-SELLING
> AUTHOR AND WELLNESS ACTIVIST.

As a woman, you can do it all! You are so powerful. You may have a career, sacrificing so much to climb up the corporate ladder. Maybe you have a beautiful family you take care of and make sure they stay healthy. Perhaps you strive for a life of success as you study online and work hard to put the building blocks of your life together. You have gotten through sticky situations without even knowing how you did it. You can survive so many scenarios, but nothing can prepare you for certain health issues that come with aging.

You can plan most of your life, but you cannot predict how aging, menopause and your general health will turn out. It's this unpredictability that terrifies most women. You're told to care for yourself from elementary school to the time you are a grown woman by eating a healthy diet and exercising so that you burn more calories than you consume. There is brief mention of a healthy gut, how you achieve it, and why it is important. This omission of the most significant aspect of your health is why women today are ill-equipped for the health tribulations that await them.

Like you, and so many other women, I had to experience a health problem before I discovered the importance of gut health, eating a gut friendly diet, and using intermittent fasting to keep a balance between the good and bad bacteria that lives in my gut. I had struggled with my weight since a young age. I was critical of how my body looked because I didn't have a healthy relationship with food. When I had my beautiful son at 27 years old, I gained more weight during the pregnancy. Postpartum, I struggled to shed this excess weight until I began intermittent fasting. My weight now was under control, but more health issues followed.

During my mid-forties, I noticed weight gain around my abdomen, and then my cycle was becoming irregular. Sometimes my period would come on time, and I would experience a normal cycle. Sometimes it arrived late and lasted a day or two. Eventually, it didn't come at all. I experienced hot flashes, and I could not get a good night's sleep. My moods were all over the show and after consulting with my doctor, she confirmed I experienced perimenopause symptoms. Around the same time, I was diagnosed with an autoimmune disease and leaky gut syndrome. It was a rough time in my life, but I became determined to find naturalistic methods to get my life back.

DID YOU KNOW?

When menopause symptoms show up, you may not be open to the change. Embracing this new chapter in your life can be difficult because the symptoms are not pleasant. Menopause signifies a decline in your fertility; this can feel disempowering even if you were not planning to have any more children. 'Once you've reached menopause, your luteinizing hormone (LH) and follicle-stimulating hormone (FSII) levels remain high, and your estrogen and progesterone levels remain low. You no longer ovulate, and you cannot conceive a child' (Pietrangelo, 2017, para. 13). This can be hard to swallow.

In a study with 1039 female participants in the United States between the ages of 40 to 65 (Gordon, 2021):

- One-fifth of the women experienced symptoms of menopause for 12 months or more before seeking medical advice.
- Over one-third were not diagnosed as menopausal.
- Twenty-nine percent did not look for any information concerning menopause until it affected them.
- Forty-five percent had no clue what the difference between menopause and perimenopause (the period of transition leading to menopause) was.

- Seventy-three percent stated they were not receiving treatment for their menopausal symptoms.

The most common symptoms that were reported in the study included hot flashes, weight gain, and difficulties with sleep. I noticed I was gaining more weight, especially around my abdomen. After researching, I found out it was due to declining estrogen levels, and this was my first symptom of peri-menopause. This means there is a direct link between menopause and weight gain. You are likely to experience this if you are not already.

CAN YOU DO ANYTHING ABOUT IT?

Menopause will arise because of your age; therefore, you have little control over it. Luckily, modern science has revealed a connection between gut health, hormones and menopause. If you support the health of your gut microbiome (microbes that live in your gut), it can prepare your body to weather the storm from perimenopause right through to menopause. Your gut microbiome is composed of various fungi, bacteria, and viruses that live in your gut and serve as the backbone for your immu-nity, digestion, mood and overall health. The estrobolome are microbes that aid in the metabolizing of estrogen. The right amount of estrobolome ensures there is enough estrogen in your system for balanced hormonal functioning.

Due to plummeting levels of estrogen during perimenopause, there is an impact on the estrobolome. The relationship between your gut microbiome and your hormones is a two-way street: imbalances in the gut can cause hormonal shifts, but the change of hormones can also affect how your gut functions. The gut not only affects your hormonal balance, it also influences the microbiome of your vagina. Menopause and the hormonal changes may bring unpleasant urinary symptoms or uncomfortable and painful sex. Instead of treating the symptoms with medications, you may pay attention to your gut diet first and improving your gut microbiome to support the health of your hormones and vagina.

WHEN YOUR CONFIDENCE TAKES A HIT

A woman's body goes through many changes from when she reaches puberty until she enters menopause. These various changes will influence your confidence and self-esteem. Sometimes these changes will feel empowering, like when you have given birth to a baby; other times, these changes will lead to anxiety, depression, and mood swings. You may already have certain feelings related to your confidence and self-esteem if you have already begun experiencing menopausal symptoms. The changes in your body can derail your sexual performance and the effect of time and aging can make you feel less confident. You may struggle with predicting when your next hot flash will occur so that you can expect when you'll be sweating. Struggling to sleep and sweating at night may leave you sleep-deprived and too fatigued to see friends and loved ones during the day.

I went through the same changes you may be experiencing. I didn't know how to deal with the perimenopause symptoms.

My clothes didn't fit right; I felt fatigued because of restless nights which affected my work performance. I turned to sugary foods for an energy boost, but this made me feel worse. It was becoming a vicious cycle; I was overwhelmed and frustrated with my body. Everything was falling apart, I thought. I did not feel pretty enough or womanly enough. I would start sweating and feeling hot when I thought things were going well. And I had also received an autoimmune disease diagnosis. This would put me in a funk and make me feel anxious and depressed. This carried on for some time until I decided to break the cycle and take control of my body.

YOUR PAIN IS MY PAIN

It can be pretty frustrating to be confused by your own body. At some point, I became curious about how to deal with my peri-menopause symptoms. After discovering crucial information about my gut microbiome and what is healthy for it, it horrified me to find out that my addiction to sugar was harming me. You may notice too that your food habits are wreaking havoc on your gut health. I know you are desperate to bring a positive change in your life. I know you are looking for an effective way to regain control of your health and improve your premenopausal or menopausal symptoms. There is hope. You can live a fulfilling life again.

This book will give you 7 habits you can use to heal your gut. They include intermittent fasting and how exercise and other self-care methods can improve your health in order to achieve the best results for weight loss and control of menopause.

When you have finished reading the book, you can apply its key points and begin creating a plan that hinges on intermittent fasting and your gut health. Implementing these methods will lead to some relief from your perimenopausal and menopausal symptoms. I use these habits in my daily life to keep my menopause and autoimmune disease under control. Chapter by chapter I will explore a variety of topics including menopause and the changes it has on a woman's body, gut health and how it affects various aspects of your health and why eating a diet rich in prebiotics and probiotics is important. I will also discuss why getting good quality sleep and living a life where you can manage stress is also a crucial aspect of maintaining your gut health.

Do not feel compelled to implement all these habits in one go. Change can be overwhelming. If you do too much at once, setbacks can be discouraging. Read this book in its entirety first so you can familiarize yourself with what *"7 Healthy Gut Habits for Women Over 40"* is about; select a habit you will have the most fun implementing, or you are already somewhat comfortable with, and start with that. The momentum from that success will propel you to take on the habits that seem more challenging to you. You can read each habit as many times as you need and skip others when you are not focusing on them.

After years of research, I understand how my gut health affects my menopausal state. Practicing the habits outlined in this book helped me improve my health status. I rediscovered the joys of life as I was free from certain pains and stresses that accompany menopause. I have been where you are, and I know you are suffering; I have written this book to ease some or all of your symptoms so that you can enjoy a high quality of life again. Before *"7 Healthy Gut Habits for Women Over 40"*, women all around the globe struggled to cope with menopause symptoms. This is the information you have been missing to make the aging process more enjoyable.

You can stop wondering how you are going to turn your life around now. From today onward, you will receive life-changing information that will usher you into a new existence. You will no longer be confused about your body, but will have the right tools to help respond better to menopause and all the inevitable hormonal changes. Keep an open mind as I reveal to you all the tips and tricks that transformed me from a flustered, overwhelmed, anxious woman to a confident, relaxed, and proud female experiencing menopause. Hang tight, because you will experience the same transformation. Are you ready?

1

EMBRACING A NEW FRONTIER— PERIMENOPAUSE AND MENOPAUSE

I was looking forward to starting an exciting new phase in my life. My son moved out of the house and it gave me more freedom. With so much extra time, I was considering traveling, indulging in art classes, and even taking up golf. I could not have predicted that my health would throw a wrench into my plans by lowering my quality of life and making me feel uncomfortable in my skin. My story is one that is similar across so many women's lives. You may even have shared some symptoms with me.

I just wanted things to get back to normal, but I could not turn back the hands of time. Every year, in the United States, around 1.3 million women experience the onset of menopause. (Dorr, 2022). What I was going through is what so many women experience as they reach their 40s and 50s. A menopausal transition is a normal part of a woman's aging process. The menopausal symptoms may differ from one woman to the next, but for most, the transition brings hot flashes, chills, night sweats, moodiness, irritability, weight gain, difficulty sleeping, and pain during sex. Your life is suddenly turned upside down as you transition from a peaceful existence to feeling like your body is fighting with itself.

This chapter outlines the distinct changes your body experiences during perimenopause and menopause. When you know why it's happening, it is easier to accept it. Ignorance often fuels fear and it causes frustration for women during this time: they do not understand what is happening to them. Knowing how menopause affects the body will give you a chance to prepare for the changes.

WHAT MENOPAUSE MEANS TO YOU

I knew menopause existed, but I didn't want to think or learn about it because to me this change meant aging and I didn't want to age. So, I waited until it hit me and I wasn't ready. It's not surprising to discover that women do not know what menopause is until they experience it themselves. No one talks about it until they have to. Did you know what menopause was before you began experiencing symptoms? Were you aware it lasts for a certain period? Have you ever heard of perimenopause? I bet you answered "no" to two or more of the above questions. Luckily, ignorance is what this book endeavors to combat.

Why Menopause Happens and How Long it Lasts

Natural menopause (the kind that is not caused by medical intervention or health conditions) occurs because the reproductive cycle slows down. This downtrend in fertility is preparing your body to stop reproduction as it adapts to the different hormones it is now producing. The menopausal transition begins roughly between the ages of 45 and 55 and can last anywhere between 7 and 14 years. The duration of this period depends on lifestyle factors, genetics, age of onset, race and ethnicity. You are less likely to conceive, but it's still possible.

How Your Hormones Change During Menopause

The simplest way to explain the hormonal changes that come with menopause is your ovaries no longer produce sufficient amounts of hormones to support and control menstruation. Estrogen levels are no longer stable; they will vary and eventually settle at a very low level. Estrogen impacts your cholesterol levels and how your body metabolizes calcium. During this transition, your body will use energy differently and the fat cells change, resulting in easier weight gain. You may also experience changes in your heart and bone health, making it crucial to keep up with your regular medical checkups with your healthcare provider.

How Menopause Occurs

When you have gone through 12 consecutive months without having a period, you are considered being in menopause (Pietrangelo, 2017). The time leading to that point, where you experience symptoms or changes in your menstrual cycle, is called perimenopause. Imagine your reproductive cycle as a smooth-functioning sports car. The car was speeding carelessly along the freeway in your earlier days. Unfortunately, the sports car, like the reproductive system, was not designed to run at high speeds indefinitely.

Eventually, your body needs to leave the freeway to find a parking spot. Menopause is the parking spot. Perimenopause is the shifting gears of this vehicle that allows you to slow down safely and apply the brakes.

Three stages define natural menopause:

- Perimenopause: the transition phase lasts until the point when your ovaries cease releasing eggs. In the last two years of this phase, the drop in estrogen levels speeds up, but you can still conceive as your periods may not have stopped yet.
- Menopause: during this phase, menstruation comes to a complete end. Your ovaries stop releasing eggs.
- Postmenopause: this is the stage after your period stopped for a year, and it lasts for the rest of your life. Some experience menopausal symptoms for up to a decade after the transition, while others experience no symptoms at all. This phase is linked to an increased

risk for health conditions like osteoporosis and heart disease.

What Is Premature Menopause?

Premature menopause occurs at age 40 or younger because of surgical intervention or damage to the reproductive system. Sometimes a rare health condition causes the onset of premature menopause. As a woman, you are born with a limited number of eggs that mature and get released through the course of your reproductive years. The number of eggs in your ovaries varies with each individual, and sometimes the egg supply runs out quicker than expected. This is a rare condition called primary ovarian insufficiency (Cleveland Clinic, 2021).

Menopause Symptoms To Look Out For

You now have a better understanding of perimenopause and menopause, and we can shift our discussion to take a closer look at the symptoms you can expect. There's a lot more to it than the infamous hot flashes parodied in popular media. If you experience some symptoms below, you might be in the transitioning phase. Your healthcare provider can confirm the onset of menopause. Symptoms signifying menopause include (Cleveland Clinic, 2021):

- discomfort during sex and the experience of vaginal dryness
- hot flashes
- chills

- night sweats
- mood swings, mild depression and other emotional changes
- frequent urination
- insomnia
- dry skin, eyes, or mouth
- digestive issues

The effect menopause can have on your gastrointestinal tract may also cause the following symptoms in relation to your gut (Nathoo, 2022):

- feeling bloated and gassy
- acid reflux
- diarrhea
- cramps in your stomach
- constipation
- indigestion
- nausea

If you are still in perimenopause, the following symptoms may affect you as well (Cleveland Clinic, 2021):

- intensified PMS (premenstrual syndrome)
- breasts feel tender or sore
- skipping your period or irregular periods
- lighter or heavier menstrual flow than normal

Besides the above symptoms, you might experience a rapidly beating heart, pain, or discomfort in your joints and muscles, headaches, temporary difficulty in focusing or remembering things, weight gain, a difference in your sex drive, and hair loss/thinning.

Experiencing some or all these symptoms signifies that estrogen production in your ovaries has declined, or there is a destabilization in your hormone levels. Keep in mind not everyone will experience these symptoms and that other conditions have similar symptoms. Therefore, the best course of action is to ensure there is no other cause contributing to your symptoms. You cannot self-diagnose menopause and it is important to seek medical advice. Other things may go on in your body you are not aware of.

Complications To Be Aware Of

There is a link between estrogen loss during menopause and several health complications that become more common as we journey through the aging process. During postmenopause, these problems are more likely to surface (WebMD Editorial Contributors, n.d.):

- cardiovascular disease
- osteoporosis, which is a loss of bone density
- bladder and bowels failing to function properly
- increased likelihood of developing wrinkles
- risk of developing Alzheimer's disease
- loss of muscle mass and tone increases the risk of falls and injury
- degeneration of eyesight, and cataracts may develop

EFFECTS OF MENOPAUSE ON THE BODY

When menstruation stops, it is one of the most noticeable effects of menopause. Unfortunately, it's not the only one. Some consequences of the decrease in estrogen are more subtle than others. There are several body functions that are disrupted by the hormonal changes. Menopause impacts the following systems:

- The endocrine system:

'The endocrine system is a complex network of glands and organs. It uses hormones to control and coordinate your body's metabolism, energy level, reproduction, growth, and development, and response to injury, stress and mood' (John Hopkins Medicine, 2019). Estrogen and progesterone form part of the endocrine system. Dropping estrogen levels may trigger hot flashes. When you experience hot flashes, you will feel a sudden onset of heat, you will sweat and feel flushed. When hot flashes occur, they can last for several minutes at a time. Lifestyle changes (such as reducing caffeine and hot drinks) and mindful meditation have been used to manage and cope with hot flashes.

- The reproductive system:

As the regularity of your period dwindles, fewer eggs are being released to be fertilized. When your cycle stops, your cervical mucus will stop thickening as a sign of ovulation and to aid conception. Expect to experience vaginal dryness and a lower sex drive. Suggestions like an over-the-counter lubricant can assist with vaginal dryness and your doctor can suggest ways to boost your sex drive.

- The nervous system:

Menopause takes a toll on your mood. You may feel euphoria one minute and then sadness the next. Irritability is a common experience for women going through this stage. Be cognizant of the fact that menopause can be a trigger for depression and anxiety and seek medical advice if your anxious and depressive state lasts over two weeks.

- The skeletal and muscular systems:

Menopause heightens your risk of developing osteoporosis due to bone density loss. Aging causes loss of muscle mass and tone; coupled with the effects of menopause, you lose muscle at an increased rate. You may also feel aches and stiffness in your joints.

- The cardiovascular system:

Estrogen has a positive and protective effect on your cardiovascular system. When your estrogen levels drop, it puts you at a higher risk for cardiovascular diseases. Lower estrogen, which increases your risk of stroke and heart attack, will affect your cholesterol levels.

- Fat distribution:

Estrogen influences fat distribution in your body. You will keep fat easier because estrogen levels decline during peri-menopause. During your fertile years, fat is stored in your lower body, making it 'pear-shaped'. After menopause, you may become more 'apple-shaped' as fat settles in your midsection due to low levels of estrogen.

- The digestive system:

Changes in your bowel movements, bloating, and pain in your gut can all occur as you transition into menopause. A decline in progesterone and estrogen may lead to slower movement of food in the digestive tract; this means your body reabsorbs moisture, making the waste dry and leaving you at risk of becoming constipated, bloated and gassy. Your gallbladder may take longer to empty itself of bile, leading to a higher risk of developing gallstones and other gallbladder related problems.

Lower estrogen levels also impact your bladder control. Menopause can cause your bladder to leak, and you may notice the leaks when you are coughing, laughing, sneezing, or working out. Frequent urination can interfere with your sleeping patterns.

The effects of menopause on your entire body may feel like your life is being turned upside down. Of particular importance is the link between this hormonal transition and weight gain. Understanding how menopause influences your weight gain can help you expect the potential changes to our digestion.

MENOPAUSE AND WEIGHT GAIN

It seems like weight gain is unavoidable when you go through menopause, but does this always have to be the case? At first glance, yes, especially because weight gain is a common occurrence during perimenopause and menopause. If you dive deeper, though, it soon becomes apparent there is more to the status quo than a cursory observation would have you believe. There is no magic formula to apply to stop this weight gain, but if you understand why it happens, you can be proactive about preventing it and it will be easier to deal with.

As you age, there are various conditions that can cause weight gain, such as certain medications and medical conditions. The older you get, the more these conditions are likely to affect your body and how you keep weight and fat. Aging and changing hormones are the biggest contributors to weight gain during menopause. And reduced levels of estrogen are in the center of it all. Estrogen is a key component of weight management, according to some animal studies. Low levels of estrogen in lab animals make them less physically active and they feed more (WebMD Editorial Contributors, n.d.).

Metabolic rate (the rate at which your stored energy transforms into working energy) is thought to be slowed down by having low levels of estrogen. There is some evidence that a woman who receives estrogen replacement therapy will benefit from a boost in her resting metabolic rate (WebMD Editorial Contributors, n.d.). This might help slow weight gain. Because estrogen plays a role in controlling body weight in animal studies, it is believed that the basic functioning of estrogen is the same in humans. Therefore, when your estrogen levels drop, your metabolic rate lowers, which affects the rate at which our body converts food into fat.

Dwindling estrogen levels may also trigger less effective use of sugars and starches, leading to weight gain. Lower estrogen levels, however, are not the only cause of weight gain during menopause. There are many other age-related changes that exacerbate weight gain, and they include the following (Stuart, n.d.):

- As you get older, you may become less likely to exercise due to stiff muscles, achy joints, and a fear of injury; the ripple effects of this aversion to physical activity cause loss of muscle mass, lower resting metabolism, etc.
- Your body will conserve as much energy as it can as you get older, which will make it harder to burn extra calories.
- Certain medications, a family history of obesity, and lifestyle choices can make your body to accumulate excess fat.

A sugar addiction, achy joints, and previous injury all contribute to weight gain, but an imbalanced gut microbiome does not receive enough attention. Our gut microbiome plays a crucial role in metabolism. Menopause has been found to change the gut microbiome, which may contribute to weight gain, slower metabolism, and insulin resistance (Becker & Manson, 2020). Understanding how the gut functions, which organs it affects, and its importance to your health can help you reclaim your life in a way you didn't think was possible.

After experiencing issues with my gut, menopause, and weight gain, I became so self-conscious about not only my appearance but also doubted my mental well-being. Once I understood what was happening to me, I became less anxious about my health. Menopause is a natural part of a woman's life, and it is nothing to be ashamed or afraid of. Use this period as a tool to reassert your femininity and the changes happening to you. Anticipate the symptoms and tell your doctor about them; I promise there is a solution, and you can cope with these changes. If you give your gut microbiome a chance to thrive, you may also thrive physically, mentally, and emotionally.

2

YOUR GUT AND YOUR HEALTH

Your gut health consists of many parts that work in unison to ensure that you have a well-functioning gut with a healthy digestive system and a balanced gut microbiome. This entire system is the foundation for your overall health because it affects your nervous system, endocrine system, immunity, brain health, etc. Understanding how to maintain or repair your gut health begins by first understanding what the gut comprises and how those various elements work together. This chapter will breakdown what your gut is, what its organs are and how it factors into your overall health.

YOUR DIGESTIVE TRACT

Your digestive tract is comprised of the mouth, esophagus, stomach, small and large intestine, rectum, and anus. The pancreas, gallbladder, and liver are part of the digestive system connected to the digestive tract. Your digestive system begins in the mouth, goes through various organs in your body, and ends in your rectum. After you ingest food through the mouth, it travels through your esophagus into the stomach where it is broken down and then digested in the small intestine. Then it moves on to the large intestine and out through the rectum. The primary function of the gut is to digest food and gain nutrients from it.

Your mouth chews food and releases saliva to lubricate the food for swallowing. Released enzymes begin to further break down the food; your tongue helps to move the food to the back of your mouth, where you swallow it into the esophagus and then into the stomach. A sphincter at the bottom in the esophagus prevents food from coming back up from the stomach. The digestion process starts in the stomach with the secretion of a gastric juice containing hormones, acid, enzymes, etc. The stomach also holds food until your intestine is prepared to receive it. There are gentle contractions mixing food with the gastric juice to create a semifluid mass called chyme.

Once chyme has moved into the small intestine, bile and pancreatic enzymes are released to further digest food. The lining of the small intestines also secretes juices that aid digestion; contractions mix the food with the digestive juices and move it along the small intestines. Nutrients are absorbed into the blood through villi, which are tiny vascular projections that have blood vessels within them. Once the food reaches the large intestine, which absorbs water, it enters the final stages of the digestion process. Feces are created, and they move towards the rectum where they are expelled.

THE GUT MICROBIOME

The human microbiome contains up to 100 trillion microbes. If the body is in good health, the microbial cells have a symbiotic relationship with the host. Microbial cell communities live in the mouth, on the skin, in the gut, in the genitals, and respiratory tract. The composition of the human microbiome will vary from person to person. The gut microbiome contains various microorganisms that control immunity and give protection against pathogens. Getting energy from digested food and strengthening your gut walls are also functions performed by your gut microbiome. There are various functions of the gut microbiome, and getting nutrients from food is one of them. Food needs to be digested in order to break down complex components so the gut can extract nutrients from it. If your diet is diverse, so too is your gut microbiome.

You are exposed to microbes during and after birth. They are the building blocks for your gut microbiome. By five years old, you will have the full composition of your gut microbiome; any disturbances will affect it (for example, taking antibiotics). The link between your brain and gut will influence how your gut functions. There's a link between conditions like depression and anxiety and gut function. The status of the gut will determine what diseases you are likely to contract. There is a lot of investment in gut research and exploring links between gut health, genetics, good health, and disease (McGill, 2018). The findings from these studies will shed more light on gut health and how the gut microbiome operates.

THE GUT-BRAIN AXIS

The gut-brain axis is a two-way connection between your gut and your brain. The vagus nerve carries the impulses between the gut and the brain. Communications also occur via 'various chemical messengers, the endocrine system, gut hormones and neurotransmitters' (Van Oord, 2019). Some of these communications are created in the gut (serotonin, short-chain fatty acids, etc.). The gut microbiome is a necessary component in the gut-brain axis. If there is a disruption in the gut microbiome, it can cause mental health issues such as autism, depression, anxiety or digestive disorders like irritable bowel syndrome (IBS), bloating, gas, and obesity.

Stress affects gut function negatively. When your body is in survival mode (fight-or-flight response), it will not prioritize digestion. Stress increases gut sensitivity and compromises the bowel function. When dysbiosis occurs in the gut microbiome, it opens the door for psychiatric conditions to develop. 'A dysbiosis can be defined as a reduction in microbial diversity and a combination of the loss of beneficial bacteria' (Humphreys, 2020, p.166). The health of the gut microbiome influences the regulation of behavior and brain functions. There is an undeniable link between your gut microbiome, brain, and gut; It can throw off your good health if these are destabilized. Treatment of conditions like IBS, anxiety, and depression is now catering both to the mind (meditation, exercise), and the gut (prescribed prebiotics and probiotics).

IMBALANCE IN THE GUT

Stress, diet, antibiotics, and poor sleeping habits can affect the composition of your gut microbiome. When I was diagnosed with an autoimmune disease, the stress made me turn to unhealthy, sugary treats. I started having sleep disturbances and my doctor prescribed sleeping pills to address them. How do you think these changes affected my gut? My gut flora became very unbalanced. This imbalance can wreak havoc on your hormones, immunity, weight, and overall health. Signs of an unhealthy gut include the following (Dix & Klein, 2018):

- abdominal discomfort caused by gas, bloating, heartburn, diarrhea, constipation
- fatigue or disruptions in your sleep
- weight fluctuations
- skin conditions such as psoriasis
- food intolerance such as lactose or gluten intolerance
- autoimmune diseases

Your diet plays a key role in the health of your gut. If you are not eating a nutritious diet rich in prebiotics and probiotics and you often drink alcohol and smoke, an imbalanced gut microbiome is inevitable. Medications like antibiotics can wipe out good bacteria, so be aware of this effect. Regular exercise, quality sleep and a peaceful life will contribute to a balanced microbiome.

Small Intestinal Bacterial Overgrowth (SIBO)

This condition means there are too many bacteria in your small intestine, and it is affecting its normal function. Something that maintains the right balance of bacteria in your gut would go wrong for SIBO to occur. This can be anything from your bile, gastric acid enzymes, or immunoglobulins malfunctioning. If food takes too long in the small intestine, it can give bacteria more time to multiply, resulting in SIBO. The effect of SIBO on the body leads to gas, diarrhea, poor digestion, vitamin deficiencies, and malnutrition.

Small Intestinal Fungal Overgrowth (SIFO)

SIFO refers to high levels of fungi in the small intestine. The symptoms of SIFO include bloating, gas, nausea, abdominal pain, and diarrhea. Candida species is the most common type of fungal overgrowth, and it mostly affects older adults, people with weak immunity, and children.

Leaky Gut Syndrome

Your intestines absorb nutrients and water from your digested food and pass it into your bloodstream. Leaky gut syndrome is a theory where your gut has high permeability and is leaking toxins or pathogens into your blood. This leak may cause inflammation, leading to diseases such as inflammatory bowel disease (IBD) and celiac disease. Symptoms include chronic bloating, constipation or diarrhea, fatigue, frequent headaches, pain in the joints, and skin problems. You may be at an increased risk of developing leaky gut syndrome if you can't manage stress, have an autoimmune disease or diabetes, abuse alcohol, and have poor nutrition.

LISTEN TO YOUR GUT

When symptoms of poor gut health occur, they are difficult to ignore. It is important to listen to your gut so that you can understand you need to take action. No one enjoys feeling the pains that are associated with poor gut health. The discomfort alone should spur you into action to find the cause. Listening to your gut and what it needs will lead to better digestion and the prevention of digestive disorders; your brain and your gut will function normally, thus supporting your overall well-being.

WEIGHT GAIN, MENOPAUSE, AND YOUR GUT

The gut microbiome plays a critical role in regulating your metabolism and estrogen production. The full effects of menopause on the gut microbiome are unexplored. What we know is that menopause alters the composition of the gut microbiome; animal studies suggest a decrease in metabolic rate and insulin resistance, where estrogen levels declined (Becker & Manson, 2020). 'Given these data, a deeper understanding of the gut microbiome's relationship to menopause-induced changes in body composition and metabolism is warranted and may offer opportunity for novel therapeutic interventions' (Becker & Manson, 2020, para. 1). Menopausal women face increased metabolic risk which is perpetuated by the changes in the gut and that is why such research is significant to this age group.

Because your overall health hinges on your gut health, there are 7 simple habits that can help you restore gut health and address your perimenopause and menopause issues. I use these habits to navigate menopausal symptoms; I got my life back by following this blueprint. We will discuss these habits throughout the chapters of this book. Implementing them can give you answers to questions that have stumped you for years, and it is my pleasure to share them with you now.

3

HABIT ONE — SKIP A MEAL

I have a personal relationship with intermittent fasting. Postpartum is a delicate time for new mothers and I had gained a lot of weight from my pregnancy. At 27 years old, I was very self-conscious about how my body looked. I was struggling to lose weight and couldn't find anything that was effective. I was always hungry. My body issues multiplied until my close girlfriend recommended skipping breakfast because it helped her lose weight. I didn't know that what I was doing was called intermittent fasting. Suddenly, I wasn't hungry anymore, and the weight melted off of my body. After two decades, intermittent fasting returned to my life once more, but for a different reason. This time, I used intermittent fasting to promote good gut health and maintain my body weight during perimenopause. This chapter explores the effect intermittent fasting has on your weight, hormone levels, menopause symptoms, mental health, and gut health.

INTERMITTENT FASTING 101

Intermittent fasting is an eating schedule when you alternate between cycles of eating and cycles of fasting. It's not about what you eat, but when you eat. This eating method has gained popularity in recent years as a weight control tool, yet it is almost as old as civilization itself. People have practiced different fasting methods as a religious ritual in Christianity, Islam, Judaism, and Buddhism for thousands of years.

During the cycle of eating, also called 'the feeding window', you can eat anything you want, however it's recommended to keep the portions small when fasting for weight loss, and to avoid snacking. During the cycle of fasting, 'the fasting window', you can only drink water, black, green, or herbal tea, and coffee with no milk or sweeteners.

Intermittent fasting methods

There are different intermittent fasting methods you can choose from (Gunnars, 2020):

- 16/8 Method

Restrict your eating period to 8 hours and fast for 16 hours. Depending on your lifestyle and life schedule, you can choose to skip breakfast or dinner. For example, start eating lunch at 11 am and finish eating dinner at 7 pm. Then fast from 7 pm to 11 am. Or eat breakfast at 8 am, finish eating lunch at 4 pm, and fast until 8 am the next morning. You cannot snack between meals, but drink as much water, tea, or coffee as you want. This is the most popular, flexible, and sustainable method of intermittent fasting.

The eating and fasting hours ratio may vary. If you're new to intermittent fasting, you may choose to start with 12/12 and build up from there. Overlapping it with your sleep hours makes it more bearable. Many women find that 18/6 is more effective for weight loss. The most extreme variation is called OMAD (One Meal A Day). You can eat only one meal in 24 hours, as the name suggests. It's one of the most difficult and most effective methods for weight loss, but it's not sustainable. It can also lead to micronutrient deficiencies.

- Eat-Stop-Eat Method

Using this method, you fast for 24 hours one or two days a week. For example, you may choose to eat lunch at 12 pm, then fast until 12 pm the next day, then eat your normal meals. Fasting for 24 hours promotes autophagy explained below, which has many health benefits besides losing weight.

- 5:2 Method

Similar to Eat-Stop-Eat, this method restricts you to 500–600 calories two days a week; they must be non-consecutive days. Eat normally for the rest of the week. It's also a flexible method because you can choose the days when you restrict your calories.

- Alternate Day Fasting Method (ADF)

This is a more advanced type of 5:2 fasting that involves fasting every other day. Another version of this method allows you to eat less than 500 calories a day instead of fasting on alternate days. During non-fasting days, you can eat as much as you want.

- The Warrior Diet Method

This method involves eating small portions of raw vegetables or fruit in a 20 hour window and eating a full meal in the evening in a 4 hour window. If you choose this method, make sure you eat a good amount of healthy fats, proteins, and carbohydrates during the 4 hour eating window. This method is for those who have extensive experience in fasting.

BENEFITS OF INTERMITTENT FASTING

Weight Loss Tool

You may think the obvious reason intermittent fasting helps shed pounds is because you will consume fewer calories by skipping a meal and not snacking. But it's not the main reason. Intermittent fasting puts the body into ketosis, and that's why you end up losing weight. Ketosis is a metabolic process, and it occurs when your body doesn't have enough carbohydrates to burn to generate energy. Instead, it breaks down fat and creates ketones as a source of energy. Ketones are fatty acids produced in your liver. Besides fasting, you can put your body into ketosis through the keto diet. If you eat less than 50 grams of carbs a day, your body will go into ketosis after three or four days. What represents 50 grams of carbs? It can be 3 large potatoes, 3 slices of bread, 5 large strawberries, or 2 cups of hazelnuts. If losing weight is your primary goal, combining intermittent fasting and the keto diet may be very effective because it helps reach ketosis faster. However, intermittent fasting alone is also very effective and has many other health benefits besides weight loss.

Your Body's Efficient Housekeeper

Autophagy, which means self-eating, is a cellular process where your body gets rid of the dysfunctional or damaged parts of cells. It ensures your cells always function at an efficient level. Through autophagy, any cellular debris, toxins, and harmful parts of the cells, like damaged molecules, are destroyed or recycled. Your body finds a balance where the cells are being made or broken down. This results in cell repair and rejuvenation. If your body lacks nutrients, it uses autophagy to supply starving cells with energy generated from the recycled components. When autophagy is in full swing, the body is better at fighting bacterial and viral infection and inflammation, which can increase your lifespan. You can look at autophagy as the body's very efficient housekeeper; it fascinates me. I think of it as one of miracles my body is capable of.

Autophagy can suppress the development of cancer cells and thus lower the risk of cancer. It may slow down neurodegenerative diseases, such as Parkinson's and Alzheimer's diseases. The advantages of autophagy include having healthier skin because cells age healthily when toxins are flushed from the body. When autophagy is functioning well, it slows down aging and promotes longevity, boosts metabolism, and supports brain and heart health, so you will look and feel better.

Autophagy slows down as we age, but intermittent fasting induces it. To reach autophagy, you need to fast for 24 hours. To prolong autophagy, adopt a keto diet, increase physical exercise and deprive the body of nutrients by fasting for 2 to 3 days. Eating garlic, ginger, turmeric, cinnamon, pomegranates, and red grapes can also help trigger autophagy.

Promotes Metabolic Flexibility

Your body's ability to use whatever is available as a fuel source is referred to as metabolic flexibility. Your body will either use food or stored fat as fuel for energy production. When your body can switch to stored reserves during fasting, you can sustain energy for longer, stabilize blood sugar, increase the amount of fat burned, and have fewer food cravings. Humans are wired to be metabolically flexible as a survival mechanism. Fasting was a natural occurrence, as food wasn't always available, so the human body could easily switch to the stored fat and burn it for energy, for example, during famine. The American diet creates conditions that suppress metabolic flexibility because a high-carb diet is the norm; people eat as frequently as six times a day and are even encouraged to have snacks in between meals. Your body doesn't look for energy elsewhere because it expects more carbs to arrive with food constantly. If you eat that way and your body is without carbs for too long, you end up feeling fatigued and craving sugary or processed food which can cause you to overeat and become obese. This diet can cause insulin resistance, which can lead to type 2 diabetes.

Intermittent fasting and a ketogenic diet are two ways to increase metabolic flexibility. With the ketogenic diet, there's a minimal carbs intake, so your body goes into ketosis and seeks fat reserves for energy. The effect occurs during intermittent fasting, as no food is entering the body at all and it burns fat for fuel.

Reduces Inflammation and Increases Immunity

Intermittent fasting reduces inflammation in the body; when inflammation is reduced, the immune response strengthens. Studies show that fasting reduces the white blood cell count and activates the immune system to produce new white blood cells, or lymphocytes, the essential component to your immunity. Viral infections like COVID-19 are overcome based on your immune response. While the infection persists, fasting is not recommended. Practice intermittent fasting when you are in good health to boost your immunity, not when you are down with a cold or flu.

BENEFITS OF INTERMITTENT FASTING FOR WOMEN OVER 40

For women over 40, intermittent fasting can give a world of benefits and can help with peri- and menopausal symptoms. It promotes bone health and relieves symptoms from conditions like osteoporosis and arthritis. Regular fasting can combat the stubborn weight gain that accompanies the onset of menopause, because it increases metabolic flexibility, as discussed earlier. The risk of developing cancer increases as you get older; for example, breast cancer mostly occurs in middle-aged women and only a small percentage of women under 45 experience it. Intermittent fasting can mitigate this risk by "inhibiting several critical pathways in the development and progression of cancer while simultaneously causing malignancies more sensitive to treatments" (Nair & Khawale, 2016). Intermittent fasting also helps you improve your mental health by making your body more resilient to stress, reducing anxiety and depression, and improving memory. The weight loss will also boost your self-image and self-confidence.

Balanced Hormones

The endocrine system releases hormones into your body to carry out different functions. Hormonal imbalance is something that you will encounter as you get through the perimenopause and menopause stages in your life and your estrogen levels decline. There are certain hormones that fasting can stabilize and this includes leptin (satiety hormone), insulin, growth hormone (HGH), estrogens (estradiol, estrone, and estriol), ghrelin (hunger hormone) and thyroid hormones. Intermittent fasting can improve estrogen signaling by increasing growth hormones. If you fast for 24 hours at least once a week, the bacteria in your gut microbiome are reset and this new balance can better support estrogen production.

Healthy Gut

When you commit your body to a fasting regimen, your gut gets a period of rest and it can boost the bacterial diversity in the gut microbiome because it changes its composition when there is no food available. Your gut has its own circadian rhythm and different bacteria thrive when you are asleep and not eating, and when you are awake and consume food. If there's no rest, some bacteria won't thrive. When you fast, you give your microbiome a chance to be more diverse as well as improve the gut barrier function. Intermittent fasting reduces oxidative stress, which is beneficial for your gut health. Pathogenic bacteria are reduced, while Lactobacillaceae, Bacteroidaceae, Faecalibacterium, and Prevotellaceae strains may be increased. If you already have gut health issues, speak to your health care provider to see if intermittent fasting is a good option to improve your gut health or how you can implement it into your life.

HOW TO START INTERMITTENT FASTING

When you start your fasting journey, it's better not to bite off more than you can chew. Intermittent fasting requires mental strength to abstain from food when you are hungry. It may not feel good in the beginning and you may be 'Hangry', but you will get used to it the more you fast. Choose your fasting method but be flexible. If 16:8 is too difficult, switch to a shorter fasting window. No matter what method you choose, always eat nutritious, whole, high quality foods to keep you satiated during your fasting window and make sure you don't overeat or binge in your feeding window. Eat plenty of fruit, vegetables, proteins, and healthy fats and avoid processed and high-sugar foods. Drink plenty of water to stay hydrated. When intermittent fasting works its magic and puts your body into ketosis, you find you aren't hungry.

Here are some more tips that will make your intermittent fasting journey easier (Vanner, 2020):

- start a fasting journal where you plan out your intermittent fasting and write down your thoughts and feelings throughout the journey
- choose the best times for you to fast based on your schedules and activities
- mindfully get through the hunger waves when they come, as hunger will eventually subside
- gradually ease yourself into the lifestyle by starting with small fasting periods and adding more time as you adjust to it
- keep yourself busy throughout your fasting period
- stay well hydrated (more about it below)
- don't binge when breaking fast
- surround yourself with people who support your new lifestyle

- be patient and give yourself at least 30 days to adjust to your new way of life

HYDRATION IS THE KEY

It's easy to get dehydrated during fasting. Many people don't meet a recommended 8 glasses of water a day even when they eat normally; they still may get plenty of water if they eat soups, fruit, vegetables, etc., because 20 to 30% of water comes from food. But because there's no food during fasting, hydration by drinking water becomes critical to maintain. You may not feel thirsty, but you may become fatigued, experience headaches, bloating, and constipation. These are the signs of dehydration. You lose more water during fasting because your body uses it to cleanse. Make sure you drink plenty of clean, filtered water. If you boil water, it becomes slightly more alkaline, and it's a good thing. Drink at least 2 liters of water a day besides any coffee or tea. It will help your body flush toxins and be in an efficient autophagy mode. I drink as much as 500 ml when I wake up in the morning, after a few hours without drinking water.

Besides losing water, you'll also lose electrolytes during fasting. Electrolytes are the minerals your body needs to perform its functions: sodium, magnesium, phosphorus, calcium, etc. You receive them with food, so during fasting you may become electrolyte deficient. A simple way to get electrolytes is to add a pinch of Himalayan salt to your water. Himalayan salt contains sodium and many other important minerals. Don't use table salt; it's been highly refined, stripped of minerals and likely contains added chemicals.

INTERMITTENT FASTING SIDE EFFECTS

Intermittent fasting is considered safe for the majority of people, but we're all different. It is not suitable for everyone, especially children under 18, pregnant or lactating women, people with immunodeficiencies, dementia, or those who have a history of eating disorders and certain health conditions. It's important to consult with your doctor first if you suspect you may have a certain health condition that intermittent fasting may worsen.

There may be some negative side effects when you fast. Some of them occur at the beginning as your body adjusts: you may feel tired, irritable, constipated, or have bad breath. If you hydrate, take electrolytes, and eat whole food high in nutrients, these side effects will probably subside after a few days or a couple of weeks. But if they persist and more side effects continue to show up (mood swings, hair loss, binging, digestive issues and worsening of any symptoms you already had), stop fasting and see your doctor immediately.

Once I reintroduced intermittent fasting into my life again, a lot of health issues I was experiencing began to improve. The stubborn weight gain that accompanies menopause was no longer a big issue for me. My leaky gut symptoms improved, and I just felt a lot better about myself after getting into inter-mittent fasting. I felt like I was in full control of my body and my gut health. Intermittent fasting could be the key to more stabilized hormones and reduced inflammation for you, too. Your body can enjoy autophagy and metabolic flexibility if you commit to a regular fasting schedule. The advantages outweigh the initial discomfort and I recommend you start intermittent fasting as soon as you can because it is a game changer. Don't be afraid to experiment, but remember to always get clearance from your doctor before partaking in any kind of diet change. The following chapter will explain the advantages of prebiotics and probiotics and why they are essential to good gut health.

4

HABIT TWO — MAKE BIOTICS YOUR FRIENDS

U nderstanding your gut and gut health is important for maintaining your overall health. Knowing what to put into your gut will help you get optimal results. Incorporating prebiotics and probiotics into your diet can unlock many gut health benefits that add longevity to your life. This chapter delves into what prebiotic and probiotics are and how to consume them to cope with aging, menopause, and other health issues. My introduction to gut health came after my leaky gut syndrome diagnosis. I knew little about prebiotics and probiotics; I didn't know what they were or how they affected gut health. In order to ease my symptoms and improve my gut health, I had to first understand what my diagnosis was and then move on to how prebiotics and probiotics could improve my situation. You may be in shortage of this necessary fiber and bacteria, but after reading this chapter, you will understand what changes to make to improve your gut health.

WHAT ARE PREBIOTICS?

Prebiotics are special plant soluble fibers that allow your digestive function to work better and aid the growth of healthy bacteria in your gut. They serve as food for good bacteria and move through your body without being absorbed. You can find prebiotics in apples, bananas, flaxseed, green vegetables, onions, etc. Products can come with added prebiotics, such as baby formula or bread, and they will state on the label they have been fortified with prebiotics. When you see any of the following terms on the label: fructooligosaccharides, chicory fiber, galactooligosaccharides, oligofructose, and inulin, then you know it contains prebiotics.

Benefits of Prebiotics

Including prebiotics in your diet will give you the benefits of having a healthy gut lining and an improved calcium absorption rate. They improve your glycemic index rate (how food intake affects blood sugar levels) and increase the speed of fermenting food, thus reducing your chance of developing constipation. Consuming too much prebiotics can lead to bloating, gas, diarrhea, and constipation so it's better to get them from whole foods along with other minerals, vitamins, and antioxidants. If you have irritable bowel syndrome, prebiotics can exacerbate your symptoms. Having small intestinal bacterial overgrowth (SIBO) means that prebiotics will not be safe for you to take.

What Prebiotics Do

Prebiotic fiber forms part of the many foods that you may consume every day. What makes it remarkable is that it can travel through the body without being affected by the body heat or digestive acids present in the digestive tract. Prebiotics work to keep your immune system strong while supporting bone health and maintaining your body weight. When you consume anything that has magnesium or calcium, prebiotics help your body absorb these minerals better. They regulate bowel movements and assist in the production of hormones that regulate appetite. Knowing how prebiotics travel through the body is important because they have a crucial function at the end of their journey, which ends in the colon.

There are microorganisms living in your gut, and they need a food source in order to thrive. This food source has to bypass digestion in order to reach your colon and feed your gut microorganisms. Prebiotics are what these microorganisms feed on. In order to have a long life span, the gut microorganisms ferment and metabolize prebiotics. The by-products of the metabolizing and fermentation process create an ideal environment for your gut health. A by-product of the metabolizing of prebiotics is short-chain fatty acids; they can increase mucus production, disease resistance, reduce inflammation and maintain the health of your colon cells. The benefit depends on which prebiotic is being metabolized or fermented.

TYPES OF PREBIOTIC FOOD

Prebiotic foods are those that are high in fermentable soluble fiber. We find the most common kinds of prebiotics, inulin and pectin, in resistant starches. The number of prebiotics you get from your food depends on whether you eat cooked or raw food. Food composition also changes depending on whether you bake, grill, boil, fry or steam it.

Resistant Starches

Resistant starches do exactly what their names suggest: they resist digestion. They are a type of carbohydrate and have fewer calories than other starches. The reason resistant starches can travel through the digestive tract without being digested is that they serve as food for microorganisms that live in your colon. A by-product of the metabolizing of resistant starches is butyrate, which has three major benefits: reducing inflammation, increasing immunity, and improving the absorption of electrolytes and water. If your gut has the right bacteria and you are consuming foods that create a lot of butyrates, your levels will be high enough to enjoy the benefits. You can find resistant starches in the following foods:

- oats
- beans and legumes
- cooled boiled potatoes
- rice
- barley
- green bananas

Your colon health benefits from having high levels of butyrate and it serves as an energy source for the cells in your colon. It reduces your risk of developing colorectal cancer, as wel as improves your colon's pH level. For your body to regulate your blood sugar, it needs to have high levels of insulin sensitivity. Resistant starches promote your body's response to insulin, reducing your chances of developing type 2 diabetes and similar blood sugar related illnesses. Because resistant starches are difficult to digest, your body may use a lot of energy to digest them. This will cause you not to be hungry and will prevent overeating.

Inulin

Inulin, a prebiotic fiber originating in plants, helps make your bowel movement more efficient and makes you feel satisfied for much longer. There are many benefits to this kind of prebiotic, such as lowering LDL cholesterol, allowing good bacteria in the gut to thrive, and keeping your blood sugar level stable. When you include inulin in your diet, you reduce your risk of developing colon cancer. It can be found in food or as a supplement. The benefit of taking it through a food source is that those foods also have antioxidants, minerals, and vitamins that also benefit your gut health. Find inulin in:

- garlic
- asparagus
- onions
- soybeans
- burdock/chicory root.

- dandelion greens
- artichokes
- leeks
- yams

Because of inulin's ability to promote bowel movements, it can reduce constipation and improve stool consistency. A study conducted over 4 weeks showed that older adults who ingested 15 grams in their life every day reported experiencing less constipation and improved digestion (Spritzler, 2020).

Pectin

Pectin is a gel-like starch that is found in most fruits. You find it in the pulp of apples and is used to make jams and jelly. More human studies will uncover the full benefits of pectin. Pectin is a substance that has anti-tumor and antioxidant properties. When this prebiotic is present, it will improve the resilience of your intestinal lining and encourage the diversity of your gut microbiome. The following foods are high in pectin:

- apricots
- apples
- potatoes
- tomatoes
- green beans
- carrots
- raspberries
- peaches

One benefit of pectin is that it decreases the likelihood of bacterial disease affecting your overall health. This occurs because pectin prohibits pathogens from adhering themselves to epithelial cells present in your intestinal lining, which promotes the intestinal immune barrier. The current studies show that pectin could be an essential dietary fiber that maintains good gut health and reduces certain inflammatory conditions that compromise your gut microbiome (Beukema et al., 2020).

Prebiotic Foods to Incorporate Into Your Diet

The prebiotics you choose to incorporate into your diet are subject to taste and availability. You can use what is available to you. You can choose to create new recipes that include prebiotics, or you can work them into the meals you already prepare daily. The best prebiotics include (Semeco, 2016):

- Seaweed
- Wheat bran
- Flaxseeds
- Bananas
- Cocoa
- Yacon root
- Jicama root
- Asparagus
- Berries
- Garlic
- Dandelion
- Leeks
- Legumes

- Oats
- Most green vegetables

HOW TO TAKE PREBIOTICS

When you introduce prebiotics to your diet, do it is gradually, as you don't want to create a change that will shock your body. Prebiotics get to work immediately and if you have overloaded your body with them, they will create excess gas and it will cause discomfort and bloating. The microorganisms present in your gut are working hard during the day because of the circadian rhythm that dictates your sleep-wake cycle; consuming prebiotics later in the day can interfere with your sleep. If you are getting them from natural food sources, then there is nothing wrong with eating plenty of fruits and vegetables.

If you have IBS or SIBO, check with your doctor to determine which prebiotics you can eat, as some will be bad for your gut health. People with the above gastrointestinal issues may be prescribed a low FODMAP (fermentable oligosaccharides, disaccharides, monosaccharides and polyols) diet. FODMAP are certain sugars the intestines cannot digest. If you have a FODMAP intolerance, prebiotics may cause you further bloating, diarrhea, constipation or gas. It is estimated that only 5% of Americans are consuming the right amount of fiber every day (Woods, 2021). When you are experiencing signs of poor gut health, you can either boost your intake of prebiotic food or take a prebiotic supplement. Pick the same time every day to take your supplement.

WHAT ARE PROBIOTICS?

Probiotics are good bacteria that impact your gut health positively; they are microorganisms and certain kinds of yeasts you can get from supplements and fermented food. Kimchi and yogurt are examples of probiotic food. Probiotics differ from prebiotics, as the latter is a type of dietary fiber, while the former is bacteria that may already be in your gut. Sometimes products contain both prebiotics and probiotics, and they are called synbiotics. Common types of probiotics include *Lactobacillus, Bifidobacteria, Streptococcus, Saccharomyces, Enterococcus, Bacillus,* and *Escherichia.*

Importance of Probiotics

The metabolic function of the bacteria, fungi, viruses, helminths and archaea present in your gut works as if your gut microbiome is an organ. Certain vitamins, like vitamin K and some B vitamins, are created in the gut. Short-chain fatty acids are also created by probiotics. For example, propionate and butyrate are some of the short-chain fatty acids produced by probiotics and they are important in keeping your gut lining healthy and to execute metabolic functions. My naturopathic doctor introduced probiotics to me. I incorporate them into my diet to heal my leaky gut, repair my gut lining, reduce inflammation, and restore the bacterial balance of my gut microbiome.

How Probiotics Impact Digestive Health

The consensus is that probiotics have a positive effect on the digestive health as they can help combat the diarrhea and their negative effects caused by taking antibiotics. When you are prescribed antibiotics, they can eradicate good bacteria in your gut. This can cause harmful bacteria to multiply and it can cause diarrhea. Probiotics can combat IBS and reduce symptoms such as gas, bloating, constipation and diarrhea. Preliminary research shows that probiotics aid in the treatment of Crohn's disease and ulcerative colitis, although we need more research to be conclusive about the effect of probiotics on the treatment of inflammatory bowel diseases (Gunnars, 2018).

How Probiotics Impact Weight Loss

A person with a normal body weight has a different gut microbiome than an obese person. Research shows that a change in the state of your gut health plays a role in the development of obesity (Gunnars, 2018). There is a theory certain probiotics aid in weight loss, but it is still unknown which specific strain should be used, the dosage, and the long-term effects. A study conducted on over 200 people who had excess fat around their abdominal area analyzed the effect of taking a daily dose of the probiotic *Lactobacillus Gasseri* on their weight. Participants reported a loss of 8.5% of belly fat in three months. Once they stopped taking the probiotic the fat they lost was regained within one month (Gunnars, 2018). In this way, taking probiotics can be a preventative measure against obesity.

Psychobiotics

Your gut and your brain are connected via the gut-brain axis. This axis interlinks your central and enteric nervous systems. Certain bacteria can influence your brain through this axis and cause disease. These bacteria are the foundation of a new field referred to as psychobiotics. Cognitive and neurological disorders may be treated with psychobiotics, including Alzheimer's and Parkinson's disease and autism. Current research is ongoing, and it is based on which bacteria this could be and their effect when interacting with the brain.

Other Health Benefits of Probiotics

Probiotics lower inflammation in the body and reduce blood cholesterol and blood pressure. For those diagnosed with clinical depression, *Lactobacillus helveticus* and *Bifidobacterium Longum* can reduce symptoms of anxiety and depression. Probiotics increase the longevity as they promote the cell's ability to replicate; certain probiotics also aid in skin health and can treat acne, eczema, and other skin disorders. Probiotics can promote more efficient immune function and reduce the risk of infections.

Types of Probiotics

- Lactobacillus: This is the most common type of probiotic, and it's found in yogurt or other fermented foods. Various strains of Lactobacillus can relieve symptoms of diarrhea and relieve symptoms of those who are lactose intolerant.

- Bifidobacterium: This is also a common type of probiotic sourced from certain dairy products. It is often used to help calm the symptoms of IBS and other gastrointestinal issues.
- Saccharomyces Boulardii: Used to combat digestive issues like diarrhea, this is a type of yeast that is found alongside probiotics.

OVERDOSING ON PROBIOTICS

It is unlikely to overdose on probiotics unless you take large doses of the supplement. Even then, you can't overdose per se, but you can cause yourself to have stomach discomfort if you take too many probiotics. Perhaps you're taking a higher dose than you should, and you are not aware of it. Gas, bloating, nausea or diarrhea are the signs of consuming excessive probiotics.

WHAT PROBIOTICS MEAN FOR WOMEN OVER 40

Because of the health challenges women over 40 experience, probiotics could be a game changer. It is always prudent to check with your doctor before taking any kind of supplement to ensure they don't interfere with any medication you are on or the condition you have. There are a few medical conditions probiotics can help to treat, and they include:

- IBS
- colitis
- yeast infections
- bladder infections
- effects of poor nutrition
- negative effects of antibiotics

Probiotic-rich Foods

The following foods are an excellent source of probiotics and you should incorporate them into your diet to improve your gut health and support your overall health.

- Kefir (fermented milk drink) with no added sugar
- Yogurt with no added sugar
- Tempeh (fermented soybean product)
- Natto (fermented soybean product)
- Sauerkraut
- Pickles fermented in brine
- Miso
- Kimchi
- Kombucha
- Traditional buttermilk
- Cheese with live/active cultures

PROBIOTIC SUPPLEMENTS

Choosing the right probiotic supplement could be the difference between optimal and poor gut health. There are various probiotics that are targeted to meet the needs of women over

40. These supplements will not only keep your gut healthy, but they will also boost your immune system. You should select the prebiotic after consulting with your doctor and after looking at all the various factors in your health. Do extensive research on the brand to ensure it is legitimate and backed by scientific findings.

POSTBIOTICS

The popularity of gut health, prebiotics, and probiotics has been growing over the past decade; postbiotics are now gaining popularity as well. Postbiotics are the bioactive by-products created when probiotics consume prebiotics. There are various kinds of postbiotics, including short-chain fatty acids, enzymes, amino acids, vitamins, etc. They are new as supplements and are not as available as prebiotics and probiotics. Postbiotics can strengthen your immune system as they can stimulate the production of t-cells, which are an essential part of the immune system. Intake of postbiotics may reduce inflammation and symptoms of IBD.

Postbiotics reduce the occurrence of diarrhea, and they also help to ease allergies. Postbiotics reduce the risk of heart disease and stabilize blood sugar levels. They may have anti-tumor properties and having the ability to help you manage your weight by suppressing your hunger. Not everyone's digestive system tolerates prebiotics, but postbiotics may serve as a suitable alternative. Postbiotics are considered safe and tolerated well by most people. Those with compromised immune systems because of surgery, heart disorders, pregnancy, children or those who have digestive tract disorders may have an adverse reaction to postbiotics.

If you want to add postbiotics to your diet, they may not be easy to find as they are new to the market. Look for products that have dried yeast fermentation, and calcium/sodium butyrate on the label. If you consume more of prebiotic and probiotic-rich foods, you can increase the natural production of postbiotics because they are byproducts of metabolizing good bacteria.

Including prebiotic and probiotic foods or supplements into your diet could be the key to promoting good gut health. It is important to know the difference between the two. In most cases, both are safe to take, but always check with a medical professional for adverse effects on your health.

Now you know what foods to eat for your gut, but there's another issue that can have a negative effect on your gut health, and it's related to how you eat. You may mindlessly scarf down food, not paying attention to the eating process and without chewing your food properly. Find out the effect of eating slowly and mindfully in the next chapter.

5

HABIT THREE — COUNT YOUR CHEWS

We place great emphasis on what and when we eat and how we cook. Do you recall ever receiving any advice on how you should eat your food? Unfortunately, the way you eat can have a negative effect on your health. In this chapter, we will focus on why you should eat slowly, and how that will affect your gut health. Mindful eating may be a foreign term, but its benefits are crucial to keeping your gut happy. Turning to natural remedies to heal myself leads me to appreciate healthy food and mealtimes more. My husband and I made it a point to find new and interesting recipes. We would set a beautiful table and savor every moment. I am grateful for my mealtimes and the meals I am eating. I used to count my chews, but it's now a habit, and I want to teach you how to do it.

THE REASONS WE EAT FAST

Do you remember your last meal? Did you scarf it down or did you take a moment to savor the smells, textures, and flavors? Life is fast-paced; you may not have time to slow down and eat mindfully. You may not have time to relax, chew your food thoroughly, and allow it to mix well with your saliva in order to boost digestion.

There could be various reasons you may eat your food too fast (Berk, 2019):

- When you dine with somebody who is eating too fast, you may subconsciously mirror their behavior and mimic their eating style.
- Being too hungry can cause you to eat fast when you get the chance to eat. Your body is trying to fill your stomach as fast as possible because it believes that you are in a survival-type of situation and needs to respond quickly in order to afford you adequate protection.
- Your body's response to any kind of real or perceived threat may be to eat quickly while you are in that stressed state.
- When you have a moral conflict about what or why you're eating, it may cause cognitive dissonance within you and lead you to eat quickly so that you can pretend it didn't happen at all.
- If you have developed a habit of eating fast, it is difficult to slow down and eat mindfully.

Eating quickly slows down your brain's response to alert you when you have had enough to eat, which means you are at a higher risk of overeating.

THE VALUE OF SLOW FOOD

My favorite dish is a classic big salad. I enjoy anything that has various vegetables in it, but that is my absolute favorite meal. I did not discover this until I learned how to slow down at mealtimes. The colorful vegetables, their texture, the crunch, and the clean healthy taste of the meal are the major highlights for me. I started to appreciate the simplicity behind a simple dish like a big salad once I took the time to eat slowly and pay attention to my meals. Coupled with intermittent fasting, eating slowly also helped me tackle the effects of my leaky gut syndrome.

Eating slowly allows food to get digested better and gives you more satisfaction with what you are eating. It is much easier to maintain your weight when you slow down at mealtimes, as your brain has enough time to process what is happening and alert you when your stomach is full, thus preventing overeating. Slow eating allows you to take the smell and sight of food in, causing you to salivate. This provides enough enzymes (emanating from your saliva) to break down the food. It will also moisten the inside of your mouth and throat to make swallowing easier for you.

During this time, your stomach produces more acid in order to digest the food you are about to consume. If you've bombarded your GI tract with food before it is prepared to receive it, you will have problems with your digestion. Food is turned into chyme during digestion, which is a mix of hydrochloric acid, semi-digested food, digestive enzymes and water. If food is not ready to be turned into chyme, it can cause indigestion and other digestive issues. Consuming food at a slow pace leaves you satisfied for much longer; eating fast does not satisfy you for very long and you can experience hunger as early as an hour later.

Benefits of Slow Chewing and Eating

There are so many facets of eating, enjoyment is one of them. Eating slowly leaves room for you to truly taste your food and enjoy the flavors. Your meal becomes a pleasant experience that brings more satisfaction when you take your time with it. When you take your time choosing your meals, you are more likely to make wiser, healthier choices than picking processed, fatty or sugary foods that are chock-full of empty calories that will eventually lead to unwanted weight gain. Eating slowly allows your brain to keep up with your stomach and stops you from eating even when you're full; you are also less likely to snack later.

All aspects of your digestion work more efficiently when you are chewing and eating slowly. If you chew your food more intently, you will produce more saliva which not only aids digestion but improves your dental health. When your mouth is full of food, it is easy for small pieces to get stuck in between your teeth and remain there, encouraging the build-up of plaque, bacteria, and tooth decay. Saliva protects your teeth and keeps harmful sugars, acids and minerals from breaking down the enamel of your teeth.

SLOW DOWN, YOU EAT TOO FAST

The Principle of Pleasure

Food can be a wonderful source of pleasure. People can avoid healthy food and choose unhealthy food based on taste alone. Just because you have to eat healthy meals doesn't mean you shouldn't make them delicious. Just the contrary; maximize your pleasure senses by finding different ways to prepare healthy meals. When you don't enjoy mealtimes, there's no reason to slow down and savor them. Instead of eating at the kitchen counter, in your car or at your desk, make a fuss over your dining experience. Create ambience by playing some music, lighting some candles and setting the table for your meal. If you want to focus on your meal, switch off electronics. If you have to have dessert, take a few spoons and savor it. You don't need to rush to finish an entire cake in one sitting; if you eat slowly, you'll be satisfied with a small slice.

Slow Eating is Easier Said Than Done

Knowing that something is bad for you doesn't mean you will get rid of it easily. If you are starving or have a fast-paced life, you grab what you can and scarf it down as you rush to your next appointment in order to fill your stomach. To eat slowly, you have to be mindful of your habits, lifestyle and the effort you put into meals and when they occur. If slowing down your eating is difficult for you to implement, there are various tips and tricks that will help you eat slowly and shed a few pounds along the way.

HOW TO SLOW DOWN YOUR EATING

By following the tips below, you can slow down the rate at which you eat to reap the benefits of a healthier lifestyle (Spritzler, 2019):

- deliberately chew longer by counting your chews and then doubling it; soft foods need 5-10 chews, medium hardness — 32 chews, and hard foods — 40 chews
- eat food that requires extra chewing, like nuts, vegetables, and fruits rich in fiber
- when you put food into your mouth, set your utensils down on the table so that you can enjoy every bite you take
- plan for the meals to take at least 20 minutes
- sip water as you eat or any other drink that has no calories
- if you feel your pace quickening, take a few deep breaths to slow your eating
- no electronics near you should be on while you eat
- be patient as it may take time to adopt this new way of eating
- practice mindful eating techniques as they force you to be present with the smells, textures, and tastes of the food.

You can implement these tips for your entire family so that they learn slow eating from a young age. It is better to start a habit when you're older than never starting at all. You notice that you felt fuller for much longer and it is easier to control your food cravings when you eat slowly and deliberately.

MINDFUL EATING

Mindful eating is a tool you can use for weight management and to improve your relationship with food. How and what we eat is influenced by our upbringing, and if those eating habits are bad, we carry them into our adulthood. If, like me, you have struggled with your body image and maintaining a healthy weight, you may not have a healthy relationship with food. I have tried every fad diet in the world, trying to lose weight, even before I became a mother. Carrying the negative connotations I had about food into my motherhood journey made bouncing back postpartum very difficult. I credit intermittent fasting for my weight loss achievements, but mindful eating, as an advanced form of slow eating, played a huge role. Slow eating is a part of mindful eating, but the latter is much more. Mindful eating has a meditative aspect to it that adds to your mental health as well.

What is Mindful Eating?

Being mindful is a meditative practice that pulls you into the present and stops your worries about the past or the future; we know mindfulness can reduce depression, anxiety and other mental health issues. Mindful eating involves focusing all your attention on the meal before you. Not only do you focus on your meal with all five senses, you also listen to the physical cues your body may give when it has had enough food. Sometimes, an emotional response to a stressful situation creates hunger pangs; with mindful eating, you will discern between genuine hunger and non-hunger triggers. With this practice, it will be easier to cope with your anxiety or guilt about food. If you are consistent with mindful eating, you will appreciate food more and notice how food affects you emotionally and physically.

Why You Need to Try it Today

A healthy diet is crucial to aging well. The food you put into your body will determine your health status or how you bounce back from a disease or condition. There are so many convenient, unhealthy choices you can choose from daily. Your life may be rushed because everything has to be done so quickly, including your eating. Being mindful during mealtimes will shift your focus from everything else and allow you to zone in on your food, making each bite and your chewing intentional. You are including your whole body in this activity, which will reduce the likelihood of your binge eating and give your stomach the chance to alert you when it is full. There are emotional triggers that cause you to eat, even if you are not hungry, which increases your risk of becoming overweight. Identifying your emotional triggers helps you not to react to them so that you eat only when you are genuinely hungry.

Mindful Eating and How it Affects Bad Eating Habits

External eating occurs when you eat because you are reacting to food-related cues, such as seeing or smelling food. Emotional eating occurs when you resort to eating because of an emotion that has been triggered within you. When someone is binging, they are consuming a large amount of food within a brief period, and they are doing it without a thought or control. Binge eating is a type of eating disorder, and it can cause weight gain. Eating mindfully may reduce the frequency of your binge eating episodes, as well as their severity. The above are behaviors that are tied to obesity and weight management issues. When you practice mindful eating, you learn the skills and tools needed to cope with the impulses that come with emotional, binge, and external eating. You will no longer be at the mercy of your impulses, because mindful eating will give you an opportunity to respond adequately to your triggers.

Mindful Eating and Losing Weight

I have tried every diet, so you don't have to. Most diets do not work, especially not for long-term weight management. Losing the initial weight is easy, but keeping that weight off is often a lost battle. 'Around 85% of people with obesity who lose weight return to or exceed their initial weight within a few years' (Bjarnadottir, 2019, para. 22). With those odds, I don't want you to waste your time with what doesn't work. To manage your weight, you need to address unhealthy eating habits such as external eating, emotional eating, binge eating and eating because of a craving you may have. Not being able to deal with stress contributes to obesity and overeating. Many studies show you can lose weight by changing the way you eat and minimizing stress through mindful eating (Bjarnadottir, 2019).

How to Practice Mindful Eating

- make sure your meals are taking place in complete silence
- express gratitude for the food you have because not everyone has this privilege daily
- question yourself before the meal whether you are hungry and if the food you are eating is healthy
- focus on how the food makes you feel
- observe the different colors of the food
- allow the aroma of the food to enter your nose while you savor it
- Is the food still sizzling on your plate? are there any sounds?
- chew slowly and enjoy the taste
- swallow only when the food has been completely chewed
- stop eating when you feel full

Why Mindful Eating is Important for a Healthy Gut

You need to put your gut health at the forefront of all your eating habits. Fortunately, mindful eating contributes to good gut health. Practicing gratitude for the food you have in front of you will reinforce and strengthen the gut-brain connection. It's important to chew for longer periods of time in order to eat mindfully, and this starts off the digestive process fabulously, aiding good digestion. Preparing yourself for a dining experience can help your body prepare for digestion; make the effort and give your attention to your meals. These practices tune your entire body into the act of eating, which can give your body the signals that food is on its way, and it will need to be digested soon.

It sounded like it would slow me down when I first heard about mindful eating. I am a mother, a wife, and a busy professional; I am often doing a million things at once. Since learning how to eat slowly and mindfully, food has become a whole new experience for me, and I have also been able to keep my weight under control. I make a big fuss of all my meals, from setting the table to the way I present food on the table. It is a sacred occasion and my family appreciates the effort too. I see food and mealtimes in a whole new light. I hope by learning the secret behind eating slowly and mindfully, you, too, can establish a healthy relationship with food.

Understanding the effect that mindful eating can have on your health status can lead to improved gut health. It takes more than just changing your diet to turn your health habits around. The way you eat has a big impact on your digestion and eating behaviors. How you eat will affect your chances of becoming overweight. Eating slowly and mindfully places the power back into your hands and changes what food means in your life. You now know what to eat and how to eat it. The following chapter explores which gut-harming foods to avoid in order to build your gut health.

6

HABIT FOUR — READ THE LABELS

The previous chapter outlined the right eating habits to promote your gut health and enjoy your meals. To further buttress good habits for a healthy gut, it is important to know which foods and products harm your gut. This chapter will explain which foods are bad for your gut as well as which external toxins, such as cosmetics and cleaning products, may harm your gut. Your commitment to changing your habits needs to be on a holistic level. It's important to look into the food you eat and the products you use. My husband and I changed our entire lives from living in a busy city to living next to the ocean. I had a slower pace of life, so I had more time to check the labels of the cleaning items we used around the home to make our living environment less toxic. This led to a deeper appreciation of nature, adopting healthier habits, and a greater awareness of environmental toxins and unhealthy ingredients in foods. Changing one thing could have a drastic effect on your health and turn things around for the better. Human beings are creatures of habit, and it's hard to accept that you have been doing the wrong thing. Keep an open mind as you read the contents of this chapter.

FOODS TO AVOID IN A GUT HEALTHY DIET

The following foods can have harmful effects on your gut, and they include (LoveBug Probiotics, n.d.):

- Sugar—sugar can cause inflammation and constipation in a high-sugar diet.
- Soy—high levels can reduce the variety of bacteria in your gut flora, especially populations of *Bifidobacteria* and *Lactobacillus*.
- Processed foods—having a diet that is high in processed foods can interfere with your metabolic processes.
- Dairy—even without being lactose intolerant, dairy can cause inflammation and intestinal disease in your gut.
- Gluten—it can cause fatigue, stomach pain, and bloating.
- Red meat—bacteria that are not good for your gut can thrive if you consume too much red meat.
- Corn—almost 90% of all corn is genetically modified, so it is best to avoid it.
- Genetically Modified Organisms (GMOs)—foods created in a lab to be more pest and disease resistant can have a detrimental effect on gut health.

- Farmed fish—the use of antibiotics in aquaculture can pass them on to humans who consume them and destroy the diversity of your gut microbiome.
- Tap water—filtered water is a better option as tap water is treated with certain chemicals that can lead to the development of colorectal cancer.
- Nightshades—eggplant, tomatoes, bell peppers, and potatoes are in the nightshade family, but they contain glycoalkaloid; consuming them can lead to intestinal inflammation and leaky gut in people who already have gut issues or who are intolerant to nightshades.
- Artificial sweeteners—using them leads to changes in the composition of your gut microbiome, causes a higher risk of metabolic disease and increases gluten intolerance.
- Pesticides — studies show that consuming foods laced with pesticide residue causes microbiome dysbiosis and affects nervous, endocrine, and immune systems.

It's best to consume these foods less or avoid them altogether.

LIFESTYLE HABITS THAT HARM YOUR GUT BACTERIA

Your diet needs to be diverse in order to increase the right bacteria in your gut. Dysbiosis occurs when there are too many harmful bacteria. This can be caused by not eating enough fruits, vegetables, and whole grains in order to allow the diversity in your gut flora to thrive. If you don't include prebiotics in your diet, necessary bacterial strains such as

Bifidobacterium will also not thrive. Consuming too much alcohol can create dysbiosis in your gut, although moderate consumption of red wine may have a protective effect on the gut microbiome.

Antibiotics are often used to suppress infections that originate from harmful bacteria. They either kill that bacteria or stop it from multiplying. Using antibiotics may save your life or improve your health, but it will have a negative effect on good bacteria in your gut; using antibiotics may be short term but the effects on your gut can last for 24 months. Smoking negatively affects your overall health and reduces the diversity of your gut flora and increases inflammation. Other lifestyle habits that can harm your gut health include not getting enough physical activity, quality sleep, or being unable to manage the stress in your life, and we will further discuss them in later chapters of this book.

HOW SUGAR AFFECTS YOUR GUT HEALTH

Sugar is harmful to your gut health, and you should limit its intake for various reasons. There are certain foods and drinks that contain natural sugar such as fruit, vegetables and certain dairy products; these are essential to good health. Products with added sugar are unhealthy because sugar has no nutritional value but contains calories and causes inflammation. When you increase your sugar consumption, you are at risk of gaining weight and becoming obese. Sugary food and drinks can cause you to feel hungry more quickly and eat more throughout the day. A high sugar/calorie diet can lead to type 2 diabetes, especially if your consumption of sugary drinks is high.

Sugar erodes your tooth enamel and can cause cavities. Diabetes is not the only chronic disease that high consumption of added sugar can contribute to. 'The results of a 15-year study suggest that people with a lot of added sugar in their diet are significantly more likely to die from heart disease than people with minimal amounts of added sugar in their diet' (Kandola, 2019, para. 33). Because of the harmful effect of added sugar on your overall health, it's important to recognize added sugar on your food labels. Other names for added sugar could be:

- dextrose
- agave nectar
- sucrose
- fructose
- galactose
- maltose
- molasses
- high-fructose corn syrup
- crystalline fructose
- honey
- corn sweetener
- evaporated cane juice
- fruit juice concentrate
- anything that has the word 'sugar' (cane, coconut, date, demerara, grape, turbinado, raw, etc.)
- maltodextrin
- caramel

- brown rice syrup
- ethyl maltol

There was nothing I loved more than a sweet treat after a long, hard day. When I felt stressed, I would turn to sugar. Celebrating an accomplishment could not happen without a sugary dessert. I justified the constant consumption of sugar by telling myself that I worked hard and I deserved it, but I wouldn't feel good about it afterward though. I would feel bloated, gassy, and jittery; the emotional guilt was also wearing me down. I knew sugar was bad, but I was unaware of how bad it was.

Research shows that added sugar affects our gut because it destabilizes the gut microbiome and increases inflammation (Laurence, 2021). Eating too much added sugar can inhibit the body's ability to digest certain healthy foods, such as vegetables. A high-sugar diet, leading to diabetes, negatively affects regulation of blood sugar. It also compromises the intestinal mucosal barrier of the intestines, which can cause a leaky gut syndrome. Bad bacteria thrive on sugar, therefore a high-sugar diet will give them an opportunity to multiply and destabilize the bacterial balance in the gut. The best way to maintain good gut health is to keep the gut microbiome balanced. It may take six months to get back to a healthy place after dysbiosis.

You can switch to dark chocolate as a healthier alternative to sugar. Evidence points to dark chocolate being good for your gut health. The cocoa in dark chocolate has antioxidant properties that lower cholesterol, maintain cognitive health and have a positive effect on your cardiovascular health. A study conducted in the United Kingdom showed that participants who drank chocolate milk high in cocoa showed higher levels of *Lactobacillus* and *Bifidobacterium* over a period of a month. Dark chocolate, because of its low sugar content and high cocoa content, is the best kind of chocolate to consume for your gut health.

WAYS TO STOP EATING SUGAR

Cutting out sugar can be beneficial to your gut and overall health. If you are having a difficult time thinking of ways to stop eating sugar, here are a few tips to reduce the added sugar content in your diet (Rowles & Shoemaker, 2017):

- Eat baked fruit, berries, and dark chocolate, as a replacement for sugary desserts like pies, cakes, ice cream, or doughnuts.
- Drink water, herbal teas, or coffee instead of sugary drinks like sodas or energy drinks.
- Eat full-fat versions of your favorite food because the low-fat varieties usually have more added sugar.
- Use low-sugar condiments that have a label that states that there's no added sugar.
- Avoid canned foods that are stored in syrup and choose canned foods that are packed in water.
- Choose whole foods like vegetables, fruits, whole grains, legumes instead of processed foods (sugary cereals, soft drinks, fast food, or chips).

- Eat nuts, seeds, fresh fruit, or hard-boiled eggs instead of processed snack food (granola/protein bars) as it may contain as much sugar as candy and sweets.
- Eat oatmeal with fruit, avocado on toast, or cheesy scrambled eggs instead of pancakes, waffles, or granola.
- Read food labels to ensure they don't have added sugar and the hidden sugar products disguised under the names listed above.
- Use stevia, or monk fruit, as they are natural zero-calorie sweeteners.
- Protein keeps you satisfied for longer; you can eat more of it to avoid sugar cravings.
- Do not purchase high-sugar items so that they are not available when you crave them.
- Fatigue can cause sugar cravings. Therefore, a good night's sleep and enough rest can help you make healthier food choices.

How to Eliminate Sugar From Your Diet in 3 Weeks

1st Week

- remove products with added sugar from your pantry and fridge
- memorize the different names for added sugar used on labels
- use sugar and honey in moderation
- have a healthy snack, like nuts or fruit in your bag, in case you feel hungry

2nd Week

- drink only water and not any other beverages
- reduce measurements for any sweeteners that you use (if you usually add a teaspoon, then add only half)
- mix foods that are unsweetened with a sweetened version (plain yogurt mixed with fruit yogurt)
- mindfully enjoy the unsweetened flavor so that your palate can get used to it

3rd Week

- plan when you treat yourself to dessert and follow the plan
- commit to eating this way for the long term
- increase the healthy fats in your diet like avocado or olive oil
- make a schedule for your meals and stick to it

Staying committed to cutting sugar out of your diet will bring you many benefits for your gut health. The logic is simple to understand, but the implementation may be difficult. Take your time and keep on trying.

ALCOHOL AND THE DIGESTIVE SYSTEM

Alcohol has become a normal part of social culture all around the world. I used to think that alcohol was not dangerous if consumed in moderation. Unfortunately, no matter the amount of alcohol consumed, it still has a negative impact on your gut health. Alcohol is a co-carcinogen that can promote the growth of tumors and inhibit DNA repair in the cells which can lead to cancer (Alcohol and the Digestive System, n.d.). The digestive system contains many parts and alcohol affects all those parts. Your mouth, throat, and esophagus have a higher chance of developing cancer because of the tissue damage that occurs when you drink alcohol. After learning this information, I decimated my consumption of alcohol.

When alcohol enters your stomach, it limits the stomach's ability to get rid of harmful bacteria which then can pass through the small intestine. Heavy drinking can cause lesions and inflammation in your stomach lining. Alcohol can delay emptying of your stomach, which can lead to discomfort. The liver is the organ that metabolizes alcohol to remove it from the body. This process creates acetaldehyde, which is poisonous and causes inflammation in your liver. A fatty liver, tissue, and DNA damage are all the consequences that your liver suffers from alcohol consumption. Alcohol that reaches your bowel over your bloodstream can increase your chances of developing bowel cancer. It is better to steer clear of alcohol or drink small amounts in order to avoid compromising your gut health. If you have to drink, choose red wine as it has less gut-harming properties and contains resveratrol, an antioxidant with anti-inflammatory properties. Research done in the UK showed that people who consumed red wine had a healthier gut microbiome than those who drank other types of alcohol. I started to enjoy a glass of red wine on special occasions after my gut was healed.

EXTERNAL TOXINS: ARE YOUR COSMETICS IMPEDING YOUR GUT HEALTH?

You're familiar with the use of cosmetics to make yourself look and feel better. I dabbled in quite a few cosmetic products, experimenting with unique looks in my youth. I never inspected the labels or scrutinized the ingredients to find out the safety of the product. When I discovered certain brands used toxic chemicals in their cosmetics, I began inspecting labels. The cosmetics that you use every day may contain products that are detrimental to your gut health; as a consumer, educate yourself and be aware of how these cosmetic products and their ingredients affect your health. Unfortunately, the U.S. Food and Drug Administration (FDA) has no authority to police the cosmetics industry and check products before they hit the market if they are truly natural or organic. There are certain ingredients that are used in cosmetics that are not safe and they include (The Healthline Editorial Team, 2014):

- Fragrance—used to make items smell nice. This ingredient can cause an allergic reaction because of the chemicals that it may contain.
- Surfactants—this ingredient is found in products like shampoo, shower gel, foundation, and body lotion; it thickens them so that they can spread easily and evenly while breaking up the oil from your skin.
- Preservatives—this ingredient prolongs shelf life by delaying bacterial growth and can cause irritation to the skin.

- Conditioning polymers—products like glycerin are conditioning polymers that help your hair or skin keep moisture. They allow water to penetrate your hair shaft.

The FDA has banned the following ingredients from being used in cosmetics because of their harmful nature (The Healthline Editorial Team, 2014):

- bithionol
- halogenated salicylanilides, di-, tri-, metabromsalan and tetrachlorosalicylanilide
- chlorofluorocarbon propellants
- chloroform
- methylene chloride
- zirconium-containing complexes
- vinyl chloride
- prohibited cattle materials

FDA-restricted ingredients may only be used in restricted amounts, and they are (The Healthline Editorial Team, 2014):

- sunscreens used in cosmetics
- mercury compounds
- hexachlorophene

Other ingredients to avoid (The Healthline Editorial Team, 2014):

- oxybenzone
- formaldehyde

- petroleum distillates
- benzalkonium chloride
- BHA
- anything listed as "fragrance"
- coal tar hair dyes and other coal tar ingredients
- hydroquinone
- DMDM hydantoin and bronopol
- toluene
- phthalates
- vitamin A
- propyl, parabens, butyl, isopropyl, and isobutyl parabens
- methylisothiazolinone and methylchloroisothiazolinone
- triclocarban and triclosan
- resorcinol
- polyethylene compounds
- retinol

Ensure that the cosmetics you choose also come in sustainable and environmentally healthy packaging. Select packaging that is airless and won't give bacteria a chance to multiply. If the packaging allows air to enter or was manufactured in an environment that was not sterile, then it may introduce bacteria that are harmful to your gut. It's not only your cosmetics that can cause harm to your gut health, but also your cleaning products.

EXTERNAL TOXINS: HOW TO SPOT HARMFUL CLEANING PRODUCTS

The most commonly used ingredients in cleaning products are Diethyl phthalate, Butylphenyl Methylpropional (Lilial), Hexamethylindanopyran (Galaxolide), Tetramethyl acetyloctahydronaphthalenes (OTNE) and Hydroxyisohexyl 3-cyclohexene carboxaldehyde (HICC or Lyral) (Women's Voices for the Earth, n.d.). Using any product that contains these ingredients is not safe for your health. Women still do most of the housework and are more likely to be exposed to these hormone-altering chemicals. To reduce exposure, use cleaning products that do not have fragrances in them or create your own cleaning products at home from safer ingredients such as baking soda and vinegar. Do some research on safe cleaning products that are available in your area.

Harmful Chemicals in Cleaning Products

Certain chemicals can be unhealthy for you and bad for the environment. Exposure to them can affect your long-term health; knowing the difference between toxic and non-toxic chemicals can help you be more discerning when shopping for household cleaning products.

- Coal Tar Dyes—found in soap and general cleaning products, coal tar is made from petrochemicals and can contain harmful heavy metals like lead. Coal tar dyes give cleaning products their bright colors but can increase air pollution in the home. This substance is classified as a carcinogen and may cause cancer. They are listed as coal tar solutions, P-phenylenediamine, naphtha, benzin B70, and Estar; check for ingredients with D&C and FD&C.

- 2-Butoxyethanol (2-BE)—reduces scrubbing effort as it is a solvent. It's the ingredient in oven cleaners, wiper fluid, carpet cleaners, and clothing stain removers. This substance is toxic and can contaminate soil and groundwater. It is listed as 2-BE, butyl bellosolve, or ethylene glycol.

- Ethanolamines—MEA (monoethanalomine), DEA (diethanolamine), and TEA (triethanolamine) emulsify ingredients in cleaning products. All-purpose cleaners, dish soap, oven, surface, glass, and floor cleaners all contain ethanolamines. These substances can cause asthma, skin and eye irritations, and tumors. Check labels for the names MEA (monoethanolamine), DEA (diethanolamine), and TEA (triethanolamine).

- Parfums—used to make a cleaning product smell better, perfume/fragrances are added to almost all products you have in the home. Products with fragrances added to them may contain phthalates, which are suspected to interfere with your endocrine system. On labels, the fragrance is listed as phthalate, DBP, DEP, DEHP, perfume, or fragrance.

- Nonyl phenol ethoxylates (NPEs)—classified as a toxic substance, NPEs are surfactants and make detergents more effective. A lot of cleaners, stain removers, and degreasers contain NPEs. It may cause breast cancer, interfere with your endocrine system, and can wreak havoc on ecosystems. Check for Nonyl phenol (NP) and Nonyl phenol ethoxylates (NPEs) on cleaning product labels.

You may not have yet developed the full awareness to guard your gut's prosperity. With the knowledge in this chapter, you now understand what is detrimental to your gut health in terms of food and lifestyle habits and why sugar is bad for you. You are also aware of the dangerous chemicals that could be in your cosmetics or cleaning product, that could negatively affect your gut health. Implementing this new knowledge into your life-style can make a big difference. Another habit that can improve your gut health is exercise. The next chapter outlines how keeping active will promote gut diversity and digestive health.

HABIT FIVE — GET UP AND MOVE

When you were taught about good health in school, you learned to eat a healthy diet, exercise, and avoid bad social habits like drinking alcohol and smoking. Now, with research and advancements in modern medicine, we are learning more about gut health and how exercise affects the state of your gut. There are certain advantages you get from physical activity that improve the effects of aging and how you cope with the symptoms of menopause. You need to know which exercises are beneficial for you so that you can get the most out of your workout. This chapter will explore how exercise affects gut health and what you can do to live a healthier, gut-friendly lifestyle.

EFFECTS OF EXERCISE ON GUT HEALTH

You may know the benefits of exercise to build muscle mass, strength, tone, and building cardiovascular strength. Being physically active has a beneficial effect on your gut health and provides three distinctive advantages.

First, when you exercise regularly, it improves your gut microbiome by letting good bacteria thrive and reducing the bad bacteria. Recent studies show that participants who work out consistently had an abundance of healthy microbes in their gut after only six weeks; if the participants returned to a sedentary life, their gut reverted to its original state in the same timeframe (Kozmor, n.d.). Exercise has a positive effect on the diversity of gut flora.

Second, because of the effect exercise has on your microbiome, it is beneficial to your overall health. Over 100 trillion bacteria live in your gut, and they are responsible for the state of your gut (Kozmor, n.d.). When you exercise and improve your gut health, you are contributing to a better immune response, which can help to keep you healthy when your body is under attack. Your resilience to disease will improve if you stay active.

Lastly, exercise keeps your body regular. You need your digestive system to function properly in order to ensure waste is being removed from your body and that the right amount of nutrients is extracted from the food you eat. Exercise helps your intestines to contract and move food along in the digestive system, reducing the chance of constipation.

There is a link between working out and maintaining good health. Moderate exercise reduces inflammation, improves body composition, and helps heal intestinal permeability, i.e., leaky gut. 'It also induces positive changes in the gut microbiome composition and in the microbial metabolites produced in the gastrointestinal tract' (Clauss et al., 2021). The effect of intense exercise, however, had the opposite effect, reducing gut mucus and making the gut lining more permeable, thus leading to a higher risk of pathogens seeping into the bloodstream. This would increase inflammation. Endurance exercise, when done in moderation, can have long-lasting positive effects on overall health.

What Research Shows

To establish a link between gut health and exercise, studies have observed the effect exercise has on gut flora. There was a study conducted on 14 obese adults who lead a sedentary lifestyle and 18 lean, physically active adults (Pratt, 2018). After collecting a sample of the participant's gut microbiome, they then got them started on a fitness routine that included cardiovascular exercise for up to one hour, three times a week, for six weeks. At the end of the six-week period, the researchers took another sample of the participant's gut microbiome. They found that the composition of the microbiome had changed. A lot of the participants showed an increase in the gut microbes that promoted the formation of short-chain fatty acids. These fatty acids reduce inflammatory illnesses, obesity, heart disease, and type 2 diabetes. The researchers then left participants to return to their sedentary lives for a further six weeks.

We Must Exercise Regularly

After six weeks of no exercise, the participants of the study showed a microbiome that was the same as the one they had before the exercise period (Pratt, 2018). What researchers deduced from this is that exercise causes a positive effect on the gut and that not maintaining a routine will revert your gut microbiome to its pre-exercise state. Further research comprising longer periods of time needs to be conducted to discern if a greater change will occur in the gut due to exercise.

Microbiome Sensitivity

Because of its high sensitivity, your microbiome will respond to various stimuli that emanate from within the gut and from outside of your body. Exercise can affect your gut microbiome, although research into its long-term effects is still ongoing. As long as you are taking probiotics and probiotic supplements, the benefits derived from probiotics will last. Exercise has a similar temporary effect where it will benefit the gut as long as you continue to exercise. The sensitivity of your microbiome should keep you motivated to carry on and keep working out.

How Exercise Changes Gut Microbiome

Exercise allows food in your gut to move faster through your digestive tract. When stool spends less time in your intestines, there is less contact time between any pathogens and the gastrointestinal mucous layer. In this way, exercise acts as a protective measure that lowers the chance of developing colon cancer, IBD, and diverticulosis (pouches that grow in your digestive tract). A high-fat diet compromises the integrity of the intestine, but if you are exercising regularly, this can protect the intestines from being corrupted by the high-fat diet. Together with a gut-friendly diet, exercise can increase the diversity of the gut microbiome.

The takeaway from how exercise affects the gut is that although more research needs to be done, current studies reflect it is good for your gut as long as you keep exercising. Ceasing your regular workouts will revert your gut to its state before you get active. Considering that your gut health supports your hormone function and your mental and overall health, it is in your best interest to maintain a regular exercise routine so that your gut is protected and your microbiome is diverse and balanced. Since exercise influences your gut, it may also have an effect on your menopause symptoms and your mental state as you navigate that time. You may even get some much-needed relief.

EXERCISE AND MENOPAUSE

Exercise might be the last thing on your mind when you experience perimenopause symptoms. In one study, menopausal women who exercised for 12 months or more reported better health overall as compared to those that did not; menopausal women who did not work out reported worsening symptoms (Payne, 2021). Participants in the study took part in various exercises like strength training, cardiovascular exercise, stretching, and relaxation exercises. The conclusion reached by researchers is that exercise should form a part of treatment for menopausal women. Working out may not lessen all the symptoms of menopause, but it will reduce your risk of developing depression and make you feel better about yourself.

Because of hormone fluctuations caused by menopause, weight gain is common. Fortunately, lifestyle factors also come into play, so it is possible to keep your weight under control by maintaining a healthy lifestyle that includes regular exercise. As you burn calories, you are not only reducing your chances of becoming overweight, but you are also strengthening your muscles and fighting against the natural decline of your muscle tone and mass. Exercise increases the rate at which your body turns food into energy (metabolism), which ensures you do not put on extra weight. Regular physical activity prevents accumulation of the visceral fat around your organs and the stubborn abdominal fat that terrorizes all menopausal women. This means you will also avoid diabetes, heart disease, high blood pressure, and cholesterol.

Keeping your body fit ensures your bones are strong and protected from the bone loss you may face as you age. The areas to focus on easing your menopause journey are your heart, muscles, tendons, joints, and bones, as well as focusing on mobility and flexibility. Aerobic conditioning is perfect to strengthen your heart and lungs to prevent the increased risk of heart disease that increases once you enter menopause. It's helpful to know which exercises are the most effective for your specific health needs, especially because you may not work out the same you did when you were in your 20s. There is always something for everyone.

WORK IT OUT

If you want to stay independent for the rest of your life, you need to make exercise a part of your daily routine. Aging comes with its limitations, aches, and pains. Exercise is something you do a few times a week in order to improve your quality of life. The normal daily activities you take for granted, such as getting out of bed, cooking your own meals, and cleaning your home, become harder to perform as you get older. With the effects of menopause and the increased likelihood of developing certain diseases, you need to develop resilience so that you can fight off anything that may come your way.

It devastated me to find out about an autoimmune disorder diagnosis; and I also had to deal with menopause. But just as I was adjusting to my new reality, I found out that I had leaky gut syndrome. It felt like my body was giving up. After accepting my diagnosis, I could not give up on myself. I had to take control of my mental state and find solutions that would improve my body. One of the best activities I used to turn my health around was exercise. I enjoy nature walks and maintain my gym membership, as it makes my body feel stronger and my brain sharper. I was grateful I already knew what was wrong with me and that I could use natural remedies to cure myself or decimate my symptoms. Now I had to choose the right kinds of activities to reduce my risk of falling or injury. But I learned the hard way that I was doing it the wrong way.

With my weight gain, symptoms, and busy life, it was challenging to keep working out consistently, so on the days I felt up to exercising, I would do long workouts. I became stuck in a vicious cycle of injuries that took a long time to heal and bursts of energy to make up for lost workouts. If you want to burn calories and improve your endurance, look into aerobic-type exercises that make you breathe harder and increase your heart rate. To keep your muscles strong and toned, strength training is the perfect challenge. Stretch exercises that improve flexibility ensure that you keep your full range of motion while balance training helps to prevent falls. The important thing is to keep a balance that reduces the chances of injury; remember to allow your body enough rest to recover between workout sessions.

When choosing the type of exercise you want to take part in, ensure that you have discussed it with your doctor. Low-impact workouts that are easy on your joints and do not involve consistent jumping or jerking movements are the best for anyone who is over 40. This is not just about getting healthy, your ideal exercises are the ones you enjoy doing so that you never lack the motivation to get moving. The following represents the type of exercises you can get started with:

- Walking:

This exercise is free and simple to partake in and you have the freedom to go at your own pace. It improves your endurance and stamina and tones your lower body. This is the perfect workout when you are aiming to prevent illnesses such as osteoporosis. The fresh air is also beneficial for your mental stability. You can walk alone or as a group. I enjoy walking alone while listening to my favorite podcasts and enjoying sights and sounds of nature.

- Tai Chi:

This workout is called meditation in motion because you are constantly moving your body slowly and deliberately, from one pose to the next, as you breathe deeply. If you suffer from any arthritis pain or stiffness, tai chi eases these aches and even improves your heart health and sleep quality.

- Jogging:

This kind of exercise will get your heart rate up and get you sweating. Because there's some impact involved, you need to wear the right shoes to lessen it or run on soft surfaces like grass to ease the impact on your joints. Keep yourself hydrated throughout your jog and don't overexert yourself; keep your pace slow and steady.

- Tennis:

To prevent disease, tennis is a good sport to take part in as it develops your stamina and endurance. Playing tennis reduces your body fat and increases the good cholesterol in your body. If you want a less intense workout, you can invite a partner to play doubles with you and give a social element to the session.

- Yoga:

Stretching your muscles allows a better blood flow through them. It helps keep your tendons, joints, and ligaments flexible and strong. Yoga is a meditative exercise that involves deep breathing and can reduce symptoms of anxiety and depression.

- Dancing:

There are so many styles of dance workouts. You can choose from Waltz to Hip Hop to Zumba to Jazzersize. Dancing has many benefits, as it builds muscle strength, improves balance, and increases flexibility and endurance. You will have so much fun dancing you won't realize the exercise you're putting in!

- Swimming:

Being in the water makes it easier for you to spend more time exercising than if you were on dry land. If you struggle with joint pain, then swimming is an ideal workout for you. There's no friction or weight put on your joints, and you get the same cardio workout as if you were jogging or cycling.

- Golfing:

When you swing a golf club, it requires muscles all over your body to work in tandem while remaining focused and balanced. You will walk a lot to get around a golf course and carrying your clubs will provide an extra strength workout.

- Strength training:

The reason you may lose your energy with age is because of muscle loss that affects your body. By using weights or your own body weight to work out, you are building muscle mass and strength. Strength training makes doing your daily chores easier.

- Cycling:

The joints in your legs can take a break when you're on a bike because they don't have to support your weight. Your leg muscles and hips get most of the action, but your abs are also involved, which builds balance, as well as your arms and shoulders. The resistance helps to build your muscles and strengthen your bones.

EXERCISE CHEAT SHEET FOR WOMEN OVER 40

Do More Aerobic Exercise

Age comes with an increased risk of developing heart disease, according to the American Heart Association (Alkon, 2018). To reduce this risk, it is necessary to do aerobic activities that keep your heart healthy. When you force your heart to pump faster, you are building up its strength and resilience to disease; It reduces stiffness and improves heart health. Doing 30 minutes of brisk walking, cycling, jogging, or dancing three times a week is a good way to add aerobic workouts into your fitness routine. After a week or two, incorporate one high-intensity aerobic exercise, one strength training session, three days of medium-intensity workouts, and one longer session of aerobic exercise. You can build up your level of endurance over time.

Build Up Bone Health

The healing time for broken bones is longer as you age. When you reach age 40, your risk of breaking a bone increases as your bones are more prone to osteoporosis due to dwindling levels of estrogen during menopause. Working out to keep your muscles strong is a good way to prevent falling or getting injured. The best workouts to improve your bone health are weight-bearing (working against the force of gravity) and resistance exercises. Using weights to build your muscle can improve your quality of life. For example, standing up on your toes and then lowering down onto your heels builds your calf and foot muscles to improve balance, thus reducing the risk of falling.

Uplift Your Mood

A study published in 2018 in the International Psychogeriatrician showed that loneliness peaked in the late 50s for a lot of adults (Alkon, 2018). And women have a higher risk of developing depression and anxiety. Exercise can combat mood fluctuations and symptoms of anxiety because working out releases endorphins and these chemicals in the brain make you feel happy. If you are feeling low for extended periods of time, you can experiment with aerobic exercise to see if it uplifts your mood. Do 30 minutes, at least three times a week, and monitor how you feel. I enjoy Zumba, core, isometric, strengthening exercises, and interval training while yoga gives a much-needed escape from overthinking. These exercises make me happy.

Combat Menopause Symptoms With Interval Training

The symptoms of perimenopause and menopause cause your body to keep fat around your organs and in your abdominal area. When you gain weight, it can increase your risk of developing heart disease, type 2 diabetes, and obesity. Aerobic exercise may not take away the hot flashes or irregular periods, but it can help you maintain a healthier weight and keep your stress levels manageable. Interval training incorporates moderate-to-high intensity exercises, alternating a short sprint and a brisk walk as an example; or try alternating bursts of power and speed with stretching as a recovery within one exercise session.

HIIT For Perimenopause

High-intensity interval training (HIIT) is best suited for women going through the menopausal transition; it improves cardiovascular and metabolic health. Blood sugar becomes difficult to manage during perimenopause and HIIT helps to lower fasting blood sugar levels and insulin sensitivity. "It also strengthens and increases the amount of your energy-producing mitochondria; increases your stroke volume (how much your blood your heart pumps per beat), improves your fat-burning capacity, and helps manage visceral (deep belly) fat, which increases during menopause" (Yeager, 2022, para. 4). Putting your muscles through HIIT signals your brain you need copious amounts of testosterone and human growth hormones; these hormones then grow your muscles, giving you more capacity to work out and live an active life.

Although HIIT is quite challenging, it is only for a short time. Examples of this type of exercise include burpees, mountain climbers, push-ups, and high knees. If your HIIT is longer than one minute, you are increasing the time cortisol remains in your body. The stress hormone does you no good when it stays in your body for long periods of time, and this may be the case when you navigate perimenopause and menopause. How you structure your HIIT will depend on your fitness injuries and fitness capabilities. Go at your own pace, but also remember to push yourself.

HIIT Injury Risks

Your muscles need time to recover after each workout in order to prevent inflammation and cortisol imbalance. Failure to give yourself enough recovery time can interfere with your immune function and lead to exhaustion and adrenal fatigue (feelings of tiredness or as if you're getting sick). When you exercise, you are putting stress on your tendons and ligaments and joints; your muscles are experiencing micro-tears in the name of strength building. You build your fitness as your body repairs itself in between workouts. Menopause can interfere with all these things and put you at a higher risk of injury during HIIT.

Form a solid foundation with some strength training and aerobic exercise. From there, you can incorporate one or two short sessions of HIIT that last anywhere from 10 to 15 minutes. Being familiar with exercise can mislead you into thinking quantity is better than quality. Do not exercise for long periods of time as this can throw your cortisol levels into disarray. Short low intensity workouts such as gardening or taking a stroll through the golf course support hormonal balance. If you overdo the amount of exercise, it will increase oxidative stress and cause an increased rate of aging. Once your fitness has been built up from aerobic exercise, then you can add HIIT twice a week for a maximum of half an hour.

EXERCISE AND INTERMITTENT FASTING

Intermittent fasting was the first way I ever felt in control of my eating and my body. Adding regular exercise was the next one. You have the potential to burn more fat when you combine intermittent fasting with exercise, which sounds desirable, but there is a downside. When you're fasting for long periods, exercise can cause your metabolism to slow down. Fasting affects your performance and you are at risk of losing muscle mass. Choose your timing carefully so that you know when you are going to work out. If you like to exercise on an empty stomach, then you will choose a period when you are about to break the fast; if you want to use food in your recovery, you may choose to work out during your feeding window.

Different workouts require different food; for example, cardio can be done on a day when you are not eating as many carbohydrates, but strength training demands increased amounts of carbohydrates. Align your workouts with your eating plan. Make sure you are eating the right things after working out so that you are building muscles and maintaining your nutrition levels. Remember to stay hydrated throughout your workout and after. HIIT requires that you eat a meal close to the time you want to work out; eating protein shortly after working out boosts muscle repair. Keep dehydration away by maintaining a good number of electrolytes and stop working out if you feel dizzy or lightheaded. The type of fast you are on will determine the exercise you can do. The longer your fast is, the less intense your workout should be. Let your body tell you what feels good.

STAY HYDRATED

A gut-friendly diet is emphasized for gut health, but water doesn't get enough attention. A study conducted with over 3000 participants in the United Kingdom and the United States concluded that your water source dictates your microbiome composition. Those who drank well water showed more microbiome diversity as compared to those who drank tap, bottled, or filtered water. Those who drank more water had a different gut microbiome composition than those who drank less water. Studies show that drinking water can influence your gut microbiome in a way that promotes proper functioning (Prados, 2022). The quality and the amount of water you drink will not only impact your gut microbiome, but also your menopausal symptoms and overall health. The higher your gut diversity, the more supported your health will be, which is essential to cope with the various changes that affect your weight and health during menopause.

Tips to Stay Hydrated

- set reminders to drink water
- keep a water bottle in hand and sip on it throughout the day
- buy a fun-themed water bottle to remind you to drink water frequently
- try carbonated water for a pleasant change
- flavor your water with cucumbers, strawberries, or lemons
- drink at least 12 oz of water when you wake up and one glass before and after meals

Hydration is a necessary habit in order to prolong your life and keep your body functioning well, as it is largely made of water. Exercise is also an important habit to keep if you want to maintain good gut health and a diverse gut microbiome. The more you work out, the more efficiently your gut functions and is better able to fight off pathogens, illness, and harmful gut bacteria. To complement the effects of exercise on your gut, you need to know how sleep affects your gut health, which is explored in the next chapter. To have enviable gut health, you need to know how all the pieces fit together and that is what I am revealing to you as this book unfolds; keep going because you've almost got the full picture.

8

HABIT SIX — CATCH
ENOUGH ZZZS

When life gets busy, sleep and good eating habits are often the first things to go. If stress bombards our lives, we don't sleep well and often turn to escapism in television shows and social media. When we are having joyous occasions with those we love, we often enjoy the good times well into the early hours of the night. An occasional sleepless night is not a problem. If you compromise your sleep night after night, it will have a negative effect not only on your sleeping habits but on your gut health as well. This chapter outlines why sleep is important for good gut health and how you can improve your sleeping habits to avoid insomnia.

THE GUT-SLEEP CONNECTION

Why Gut Health is Crucial for Good Sleep

Maintaining a healthy gut flora ensures that other aspects of your health, such as your sleeping patterns, remain in balance. 'New studies out of Japan suggest that the connection between gut health and the mind is so strong that it can actually impact our sleep each night' (Slumber Yard Team, 2021). Bad bacteria may reduce serotonin in the gut. As a hormone, serotonin levels in the brain influence your sleep-wake cycle. It means if there is an alteration in the gut flora because of a change in diet, or other factors, it may lead to difficulty sleeping.

Brain-Gut Axis

There are certain cues that affect sleep, such as your circadian rhythm, which are biological processes based on your internal clock and follow a 24-hour cycle. The sleep-wake cycle is a circadian rhythm and anything that destabilizes it will disrupt your sleep. According to research, your gut microbiome influences a variety of bodily functions, including your cognitive function, formulation of memories, development of your brain, mental health, and circadian rhythm. The brain-gut axis is a network that comprises the circulatory system and vagus nerve, which connects brain function to your intestinal metabolism.

Because of the brain-gut axis functions, a simple solution to sleeping problems could be changing your diet and making it gut-friendly. Over-the-counter medications or prescribed sleeping pills are the fastest solution to insomnia, but they often have negative side effects on long-term sleeping patterns and your gut flora. Instead of turning to medication first, you could attempt balancing your gut health through a gut-friendly diet as this is a more natural treatment that has no side effects, unlike sleeping medications that can cause gastrointestinal distress and drowsiness even after waking up.

Diet and How it Affects Your Body's Neurotransmitters

To get quality sleep every night, your gut needs to have a healthy microbiome with the right levels of good bacteria. Having the right neurotransmitters present in the gut is also crucial to good quality sleep. There are different neurotransmitters that can affect your sleep; they work together to create a hormonal balance that encourages a good night's rest.

Serotonin

Serotonin is a hormone that delivers signals between nerve cells, and a majority of the serotonin lives in your gut. It helps maintain your sleep, but serotonin can also be responsible when you cannot fall asleep. Without serotonin, your body cannot produce melatonin from your pineal gland, which your body needs to recognize when it's time to sleep or wake up. Serotonin is also responsible for stabilizing your moods and keeping depression and anxiety at bay. It also helps heal the body.

Dopamine

Dopamine is a neurotransmitter that sends signals to and from nerve cells. In terms of digestion, dopamine helps regulate the release of insulin from the pancreas; dopamine also influences how food moves through the small intestine and colon; and it keeps you alert and awake. A study conducted in 2012 showed that a lack of sleep reduces the number of dopamine receptors, which resulted in drowsiness and trouble staying awake (Vandergriendt, 2020).

Melatonin

When it gets dark, your brain produces melatonin in response to the lack of light. Melatonin regulates your circadian rhythm and maintains your sleep-wake cycle. Being exposed to light at nighttime can stop the production of melatonin, which can disrupt your sleep-wake cycle. As this hormone responds to darkness, it is essential to keep your internal clock regulated so that your body knows when to rest and when it should be alert and awake.

GABA

GABA stands for gamma-aminobutyric acid. It is an inhibitory neurotransmitter, meaning that it blocks impulses between nerve cells. Known to prevent seizures, when GABA attaches to GABA receptors, it is also responsible for easing feelings of stress, anxiety, and fear. A study conducted in 2018 on 40 participants, who took 300 mg of GABA one hour before bedtime, showed that they fell asleep faster than the participants who were given a placebo; their quality of sleep also improved up to four weeks after taking treatment (Healthline Medical Network, 2018).

Your diet has a critical impact on these neurotransmitters. Keeping your gut healthy encourages the right levels of these hormones to be present within the body. If these hormones are out of balance, it will not only impact your sleep, but also your ability to think, feel, and function. When your sleep-wake cycle is disrupted because of this hormonal imbalance, you are at risk of experiencing low-quality sleep or even insomnia.

Coping With Stomach Discomfort During Sleep

Make sure mealtimes occur well before bedtime and you can prevent digestive issues that may culminate in abdominal pain. Eating right before going to bed means that the digestion process will happen while you are horizontal in your bed. If there is too much gas in your digestive system, it can cause bloating discomfort and distention. You can reduce the amount of air you swallow by taking smaller bites and chewing them for much longer; avoid food that causes you gas. Acid reflux is another cause of abdominal pain at night; it occurs when acid travels back into the food pipe and causes a burning sensation, gas, nausea, vomiting, bloating, and a sore throat. Drinking too much alcohol, over-eating close to bedtime, lying down after meals, being overweight, and spicy, fried or high-fat foods can cause acid reflux. To prevent acid reflux, keep your weight healthy, eat a healthy diet, avoid smoking, and wait at least one hour after meals before lying down.

The Connection Between Sleep and Your Stomach

The relationship between your gut and the quality of your sleep goes both ways. Poor gut health can cause issues with your sleep cycles in the same way poor quality sleep can negatively affect your gut health. If you are not getting enough sleep, the levels of cortisol in your body stay high. When cortisol is coursing through your body, digestion and gut function are not prioritized. This leaves your gut open to the risk of developing dysbiosis and reduces bacterial diversity. Lack of sleep also reduces the amount of melatonin and prolactin, the hormones that are crucial in maintaining good bacteria levels in the gut and proper digestion. Without these necessary hormones that aid digestion, your gut health will be negatively affected.

Poor sleeping patterns can also lead to poor dietary choices that can wreak havoc on your gut health. Lack of sleep can cause you to feel hungrier than usual and increase your appetite. You may think taking bigger bites and chewing your food less to satiate this hunger faster. The fatigue that comes with a low-quality sleep cycle can cause you to crave high-fat, processed, or sugary foods in order to boost your energy levels. If you're not getting enough sleep, you won't have the energy to prepare gut-friendly meals and may choose convenience over health. Having one or two terrible nights does not mean your gut health will suffer, but if your sleep issues are persisting over a few weeks, it may have a detrimental impact on your long-term gut health.

SLEEPLESS NIGHTS AND HOW THEY AFFECT WOMEN OVER 40

In order to age well, you need to get sufficient amounts of quality sleep. Lack of sleep can cause inflammation in your heart, joints, muscles, and pancreas. This can add to the mounting health issues you may already experience because of menopause. Sleep is restorative and allows muscle repair and tissue growth. If you are lying awake between the hours of two and four AM, this release of restorative hormones does not happen, and your body cannot heal itself or repair any cells or muscle tissue. Sleepless nights can affect all aspects of your health and compromise sufficient functioning of the bodily functions that support your overall health.

Women going through perimenopause and menopause have reported experiencing trouble sleeping. In a study conducted by the Center for Disease Control and Prevention, 20% of the participants, aged between 40 and 59, reported having trouble falling asleep four or more nights a week (WebMD Editorial Contributors, n.d.-b). Sleep issues may prevail even in women who are postmenopausal. The sleepless nights often happen because of the symptoms of perimenopause or menopause, such as hot flashes and night sweats. Mild depression caused by sudden mood changes, or life changes like children leaving for college, may lead to increased anxiety and insomnia.

There are various causes that could contribute to impaired sleep during a woman's midlife. Estrogen helps maintain muscle tone in a person's upper airways; reduced estrogen levels may increase your risk of developing obstructive sleep apnea. With age comes an increased risk of insomnia and restless leg syndrome, which can disrupt falling asleep. The risk of developing chronic illnesses increases. The medications to treat these long-term illnesses can interfere with sleep, increasing the risk of insomnia and causing frequent urination at night time. Although these several factors can cause sleep disruptions, there are various ways you can mitigate them in order to receive good quality sleep every night and to support your gut health.

FALL ASLEEP QUICKLY

As you get older, good health becomes more important. Good health is a symphony of various aspects, like a good diet, exercise, and a good night's rest. If one is compromised, it throws the entire orchestra out of tune. Experiencing aging, perimenopause or menopause does not doom you to never sleep well again. Your body needs six to eight hours of sleep every night in order for various physical and mental processes to regulate good health. If you have been experiencing issues with your sleeping patterns, try the following tips to improve your sleep quality:

- Take a warm bath or shower before bed to promote relaxation and sleepiness.
- Lower the thermostat to 65 to 68 degrees Fahrenheit (18 to 20 Celsius) and consider opening a window to promote good air flow.
- Try cardiovascular/aerobic exercise, strength training, high-intensity exercise, or yoga as these types of

exercise ease symptoms of anxiety/depression, promote restful sleep, and boost good moods.

- Exercise earlier in the day so that your workout does not make you too alert, interfering with your bedtime.
- Practice meditation as it promotes better quality sleep; most meditation techniques involve deep breathing in a quiet comfortable place to ground you in the present moment.
- Use the 4-7-8 method of meditation that has a tranquilizing effect. You begin by sitting comfortably with your back straight and your tongue resting behind your top row of teeth. Say 'whoosh' as you breathe out, then breathe in through your nose for four seconds; hold your breath for seven seconds. Say 'whoosh' as you exhale for eight seconds.
- Wake up and go to bed at the same time every day.
- Avoid any electronics for two hours before bedtime as blue light emitted by TVs, tablets, and phones can interfere with your sleep cycle.
- Have a bedtime routine to regulate your body clock and train it to know when it is time for bed.
- Make a list of things you are grateful for; write down things you achieved that day, and those you want to do the next day.
- Try using a weighted blanket and a weighted eye pillow.

The Military Method

The US military developed this method to help navy pilots fall asleep within two minutes (Breus, 2022). This is how you do it:

- relaxing your facial muscles
- relaxing and lowering of shoulder muscles
- letting your hands fall to your side
- relaxing your chest while you exhale
- relaxing the muscles in your legs
- envision a relaxing scene in your mind and hold that image for 10 seconds
- repeat "don't think" for 10 seconds

Sleep specialists say there is no standard time to fall asleep. If you suspect it is taking a long time, take note if you also experience fatigue during the day or struggle to wake in the morning. If, besides the above symptoms, you experience difficulty concentrating, irritability, moodiness, anxiety, or depression, you may benefit from seeking medical advice to see if there are other underlying causes that prevent you from falling asleep quickly.

STAYING ASLEEP

Your sleep issues may not just revolve around dozing off, they may also have something to do with your inability to stay asleep. There are several strategies you can integrate into your daily routine to ensure that you sleep for long enough that your body does what it needs to do to repair cells and maintain a balanced gut flora.

Avoid Drinking Alcohol

In times of stress, you may turn to alcohol to calm your nerves and relax you. You can feel the relaxing effects of alcohol shortly after consuming it and it can even make you feel drowsy. It may be effective at getting you to sleep, but it will not keep you asleep. Alcohol will lead to restlessness and fragmented sleep. Avoid drinking alcohol for at least four hours or more before going to bed to give your body enough time to metabolize it and flush it out.

Avoid Caffeine After 12 p.m.

Coffee, energy drinks, black tea, and soda contain caffeine. Caffeine is one of the fastest ways to get a boost in energy and concentration. That is why so many people start their day with a cup of coffee. Unfortunately, if you drink caffeine in the afternoon, it can interfere with your sleep cycle, thus it is best not to consume it after 12 p.m.

Do Not Smoke

Smoking is a habit that can cause several health complications, including addiction, cardiovascular disease, lung disease, and various cancers. Once you get addicted to smoking, the cravings can hit you during sleep, causing you to wake in the middle of the night. Kick this bad habit to avoid sleep disruptions.

Avoid Meals and Drinks Before Bedtime

It's best to eat a few hours before you head to bed. This allows your digestive functions to happen while you are upright, reducing the likelihood of nocturnal heartburn or acid reflux. If you fill up on liquids before bedtime, it is likely that the urge to urinate will hit in the middle of your sleep, forcing you to wake to empty your bladder. Any drinking or eating should occur two to three hours before bedtime.

Exercise Earlier in the Day

Exercising earlier in the day not only allows you to fall asleep quickly, but ensures you stay asleep throughout the night. Exercise perks you up and gets your blood pumping, delivering oxygen to your brain and muscles so that they can keep going. If you're trying to wind down, this isn't good for you. Avoid any moderate to vigorous physical activity before bedtime.

Avoid Napping

Sometimes a leisurely nap in the afternoon feels like the perfect remedy to get your energy levels back up again. Unfortunately, napping can be the reason you can't stay asleep at night. Keep your naps earlier in the day and not over 20 minutes.

Reduce Light

Switch off all screens for two to three hours before bedtime to help you stay asleep throughout the night. Electronics emit blue light that interferes with concentration and sleep cycles. You could try to use a red bulb in your room or install curtains to block out the natural light that comes early in the morning. Another way to combat the insomnia-inducing effect of blue light is to use blue light blocking glasses as they allow the release of melatonin which keeps your sleep cycle on schedule, thus reducing insomnia, jet lag, and delayed sleep-phase disorder (Hester et al., 2021).

If you introduce these strategies one by one, the change is not overwhelming. Starting a sleep journal to note the effects these strategies are having can be helpful in tracking your progress as you improve your sleeping habits. It would be interesting to see how these changes also affect your gut and if they improve any of your gastrointestinal issues. If your sleep issues have escalated to where you are struggling with insomnia, there are various treatments that you can try before you turn to pharmaceuticals.

NATURAL REMEDIES FOR INSOMNIA

Insomnia is a sleeping disorder that negatively affects how and when you sleep. By getting to its root cause, you can improve insomnia by changing sleeping, eating, or stress-coping habits. Long-term insomnia is when you have had trouble sleeping for over 3 months and short-term insomnia lasts less than three months. Symptoms of insomnia include difficulty falling asleep, fragmented sleep, lying awake at night, waking up early and being unable to return to sleep, fatigue during the day, and inability to concentrate.

Besides menopause and poor gut health, causes of insomnia vary from stress and anxiety to jet lag or working different shifts. Sleeping in a noisy place, in a room that is too cold or hot, or on an uncomfortable bed can also lead to insomnia. Partaking in recreational drugs, alcohol, nicotine, or caffeine can exacerbate any sleep difficulties you are experiencing. You can try a variety of natural methods in order to tackle your insomnia (Alternative Treatments for Insomnia, n.d.):

- Acupuncture:

Ancient Chinese medicine recommends acupuncture as a treatment for insomnia. The practice involves using fine needles and inserting them into specific acupuncture points in the skin to improve certain functions in the body. Research shows that acupuncture improves sleep quality in individuals who have insomnia.

- Herbs:

Herbal remedies have been used for centuries to help with insomnia. Before taking herbal supplements, ensure you have the approval of your doctor in case they interfere with any medication you are already taking. Herbs such as chamomile, valerian root, ashwagandha, kava, hops, passion flower, and lemon balm have been shown to improve sleep duration and quality.

- Relaxation and Mindful Meditation:

Tension can build up in your muscles and stressful thoughts can manifest as tension in the body. Meditation and being mindful can help relax your muscles and your mind.

- Melatonin:

As mentioned earlier, melatonin is a necessary hormone in regulating your sleep-wake cycle. Seek medical advice before taking this supplement as research into the right doses is still underway. Take it before bedtime as it will reduce disturbances in sleep and help you fall asleep faster.

- Sleep hypnosis:

You can choose to be hypnotized by a licensed professional. They will guide you toward better sleeping patterns by getting you into a trance-like state, then suggesting better sleep habits.

- CBD and cannabis:

Cannabidiol (CBD) is a compound found in cannabis that does not have a psychoactive impact like tetrahydrocannabinol (THC). CBD may improve sleep quality, but we need more research to understand its long-term effects.

Making use of these natural remedies can give you much-needed relief if your sleep issues are not that intense. We can use them as complementary treatments alongside pharmaceutical prescriptions. Eating a gut-healthy diet and avoiding harming food is obvious when speaking about improving your gut health, but I'm sure you never would have imagined that sleep can affect your gut health and vice versa. As you age, you will grapple with various sleep issues that perimenopause and menopause may exacerbate. Deal with them as soon as they come up so that they do not turn into serious long-term gastrointestinal problems.

Sometimes being a middle-aged woman comes with sleepless nights, and that may be considered normal. I still have occasional moments of insomnia, but they do not torment me as much any more. With the use of natural remedies (CBD oil, melatonin, and magnesium), I successfully manage my sleep and minimize insomnia and I don't need sleeping pills anymore. I love my weighted blanket as its gentle pressure on my body makes me feel cozy and calm. I developed a habit of following a nighttime routine, which includes planning the next day, writing in my journal, and meditating. Many before you have navigated these waters and many after you will survive them. You can get through this as long as you understand how sleep affects your gut and how your gut affects your sleep. Even if you are struggling to fall asleep or stay asleep, you can improve your sleep quality just like I did if you follow the tips in this chapter. Good gut health requires maintaining an overall health status that is devoid of stress, as anxiety and depression can wreak havoc on your gut microbiome. If you want to know the true effect of stress on your gut, read the following chapter and find out how crucial stress management is in maintaining balanced gut flora.

HABIT SEVEN — TAKE A BREATHER

The way you live your life will influence your health. If you live mindfully, you will cope with whatever stress life throws at you. This is easier said than done. The world is stressed out more than ever. You've already been worrying about your health, your finances, the future of your career, your love life, and the well-being of your family. On a daily or weekly basis, there is an unpredictable source of stress. Navigating a world post-pandemic, where inflation is on the rise, has also increased the worries we already had. The uncertainty that is faced in today's world may cause your stress levels to rise.

Stress is something that affects your physical body and mental state negatively. If you allow stress to control your reactions and emotions, it can have a negative effect on your gut. It is important to not only eat a healthy diet for your gut, exercise and sleep well, but to manage the stress in your life so that it does not interfere with your gut health. Menopause also affects your gut health; all these different factors can mess with the equilibrium of your gut microbiome, so it is important to stay on top of your stress. There are various methods that you can use in order to keep your stress levels under control and this chapter breaks them down so that they equip you to deal with any stressful situation. Using the tools that I give you will ensure you can manage your stress and reduce imbalanced bacteria in your gut.

STRESS MANAGEMENT

Long walks on the beach have done wonders for my mental health. When the weather is good, I walk barefoot two to three times a week. The sound of the waves crashing on the shore calms my nerves. Because of the changes menopause brings, I pay extra attention to my thoughts and self-care routine. The hormonal changes you experience with perimenopause and menopause affect your mental health. Disturbances in sleep are common during menopause, and lack of sleep can exacerbate irritability and anxiety and lead to poor concentration. Some of the other symptoms that may affect your mental state include:

- feeling anxious
- loss of self-esteem, confidence, and memory
- feeling angry, sad, or depressed
- losing your train of thought

Going through these emotions, coupled with the changes occurring in various areas of your life, can make you feel overwhelmed. The mental effects of menopause can have a significant impact on your life in the same way as the physical ones. Because of the mental effects of menopause, you need to discern how you feel and when you may need some professional help with coping.

There are so many physical changes that can throw you off balance. It requires a lot of time and patience to navigate your "new" self. Relating with other women who also experience menopause may give you a well-deserved opportunity to vent about what you are experiencing. You can find a community in your area or online that will support you. Taking time for yourself can help you replenish your mental strength when you feel emotionally drained.

It is important to understand how menopause can influence your mental well-being and add to your everyday stress. Therefore, it is also important to monitor your moods and emotional state so that you can notice when it becomes a more serious mental condition that may need medical attention. Stress throws your gut off, which will destabilize your overall health. Before we can explore tips for managing stress, we should first discuss how stress affects your gut so that you can understand what happens if you don't manage your stress levels.

How Stress Affects Your Gut

Stress can have multiple effects on your gut. Stressful life events can start various digestive problems or make the symptoms worse; IBS, IBD, gastroesophageal reflux disease (GERD), and peptic ulcer disease are such conditions that stress can exacerbate. A stressful event can influence your gut functions long after it has passed. Being in a stressed state may cause you to use alcohol or food in order to cope, which can also throw your gut off balance. Stress may cause your bowels to become loose, which is why you may experience diarrhea after getting some distressing news; or stress can delay the movements in your digestive system and cause constipation. The effects are subjective, but this may cause abdominal pain and disruption in your bowel movements.

According to research, relapses in IBD may be caused by chronic stress, depression, and difficult life events that cause distress and sadness. A study involving 600 people showed their IBS would have been reduced or prevented if they could handle stress better. 'Those with higher levels of perceived stress, anxiety, and negative illness beliefs at the time of infection were at a greater risk to develop IBS' (GIS, 2007, para. 4). Research also further shows that patients with GERD, who already struggle with chronic anxiety, will have worsening symptoms if they are experiencing stress. It seems as if their outlook on life affected how they experienced their symptoms. There is also evidence to suggest that if your body is in a constant state of stress, it aggravates inflammation in your mucosal lining; this means your digestive juices may end up irritating the stomach lining beneath (GIS, 2007).

From the conclusions above, stress has a negative impact on your gut functioning. When your body is responding to either external or internal stress, it releases cortisol and goes into fight-or-flight mode. During this state, certain functions in the brain and the gut are shut down because your body thinks you are in survival mode. Your gut will not function well and oxygen will be diverted from your brain and into your muscles so that you can avoid the perceived danger. Imagine being in the flight-or-fight mode for extended periods of time. Reducing the effects of stress on the gut should be a priority so that you can also navigate through menopause without affecting your mental well-being or your gut health. It's a balancing act and there are some things you can do to reduce your stress and maximize your overall health.

TIPS TO REDUCE STRESS IN WOMEN OVER 40

Exercise

Exercise has many benefits, including improved moods, reduced stress, and better sleeping habits. There are many ways you can exercise depending on your physical ability. You should push yourself during your sessions so that you can build back any lost muscle mass and strength, but do not go beyond your limits. If you feel a sharp pain at any point or extreme discomfort, please stop the workout immediately. Get clearance from your doctor for what you can and cannot do. Safety comes first so that you can avoid injury as it also will stress you out. Recovery times after an injury increase the older you get, so exercise safely to maximize your benefits.

Sleep Well

Sleep allows your cells to repair themselves; cellular energy is restored, and hormones and proteins are released by your body during sleep. Your body is resting during sleep and the functions are running in the background. Your brain is lighting up, it is processing new information gained during the day, and eliminating toxic waste. The nerve cells are busy communicating so that they can be the backbone of your brain function. Your body needs to recover from the effects of stress, and it accomplishes it with a good night's sleep. Develop a relaxing bedtime routine so that you can reap all the health benefits of getting enough quality sleep.

Maintain a Reliable Support System

To reduce your stress, it may be beneficial to join a community that does something you enjoy. A religious organization like a church is a safe haven for many women. Others enjoy art clubs or a sewing circle. When you join a group of people that makes you feel valued, supported, and loved, you will feel a sense of security, warmth, and community. Try to explore what your interests are and join like-minded people. You can choose to rely on your family and friends for support. It doesn't matter who it is, but maintaining these relationships can help you discharge any stress you may be experiencing.

Eat Healthy Foods

Sometimes, to cope with stress, we turn to unhealthy habits to help us cope. You may be a smoker, a drinker, or a comfort eater. Nicotine and all the harmful toxins in cigarettes will make the effects of stress worse on the body. The same is true for alcohol; reliance on alcohol to calm your anxiety is never a good idea. Try to avoid sugary, fatty, or unhealthy food to calm your stress. Your body needs to be fit enough to combat the negative effects of stress, so use food to strengthen your body. Eat a nutritious protein-based diet that includes fruit, vegetables, lean protein, whole grains, and healthy fats.

Maintain a Positive Attitude and Release Negativity

Perspective can determine how you respond to certain situations. Take a step back when something unfortunate happens. observe it as a neutral event because everything in life is neutral; it's how you react to this event that will determine whether it is good or bad. Accepting people as they are will also help you release the negativity; you will no longer have unrealistic expectations of people.

There are many things that may happen you may deem inconvenient or very upsetting. If you get a flat tire on the way to work, try not to worry about the financial and emotional issues; decide to have some quiet time before help arrives. Find the grace to accept the things that are out of your control. You can meditate, catch up on your journaling, or call a friend. Always look for the silver lining and don't take random events personally. Life's not out to get you. Things will work out in the end.

Help Others

Stress can keep you consumed in your life as you try to figure out how to sort yourself out. Instead of keeping yourself intertwined in your own matters, you can commit to helping those in your community that may be in need. It can give you a new purpose and discharge stress when you remove the focus from yourself and your problems. Seeing what others are going through will bring gratitude; you may realize how fortunate you are not to be going through what others are experiencing.

Take Up a New Hobby

Keep your mind open to new and challenging activities, as they will keep your mind fresh. You will not feel overwhelmed by your worries when you are enthralled by a new hobby or an unfamiliar activity. Being present in the moment helps reduce stress and anxiety. Your mind will not worry about the future or the past when you are preoccupied with your fingering as you learn to play the guitar or when you're obsessed with all the variations in colors in your oil painting class. Getting your creative juices flowing will help you cope with stressful scenarios in your life.

Become More Assertive

It is in your nature to react to external stimuli. You can react to a traffic jam and being late for work by grinding your teeth and screaming through the window. It is possible to return a rude comment from a family member with a disrespectful one. It's easy to become aggressive when you feel attacked. You become defensive, passive-aggressive, or angry. Reacting in this way may contribute to higher stress levels, so instead of behaving in this way, you could learn to assert how you feel and express your beliefs and opinions surrounding the situation calmly.

Just Relax

Before I learned how to cope with stress, I was always in a rush. I worried about my responsibilities at work and at home, and I was anxious I may forget something. It was always 'rush-rush-rush' with me. I never gave myself time to relax, and this made me feel more stressed out. I thought I was wasting time when I was relaxing because I could do something productive instead. Relaxing is productive because it replenishes your mental vitality and physical strength. You cannot help others or be of use to anyone when you are depleted. Learn how to meditate or take yoga classes. Listen to some classical music to unwind and release any tension you may be carrying.

MEDITATION FOR GUT HEALTH: HOW MEDITATION HEALS THE GUT

Your gut is connected to many neurotransmitters, electrical impulses, and hormones, making it capable of doing more than just digesting food. It works similarly to the brain because your gut has a network that dictates the levels of inflammation and your immune system. Stress could be the reason that, after switching to a healthier diet, your gut issues do not subside. Thus, in order to get a handle on your gut health, address how you manage stress and your emotions.

When you are experiencing a stressful event, it alters your gut microbial population. This affects neurotransmitters that regulate the gut barrier function. Meditation is one of the best ways to handle stress. As you meditate, your stress will be reduced and your gut will suppress chronic inflammation and maintain a healthier gut barrier function. This is why it is crucial to incorporate meditation into your daily routine to support your overall health. Current research suggests meditation should be integrated into your health regimen, although more research needs to be done into the full effects of meditation on gut health (Househam et al., 2017).

Incorporating Meditation Into Your Life

When you are still new to the idea of meditation, it's hard to sit quietly for long periods of time, so I recommend you start small and build up from there. You could begin by appreciating a sunrise or sunset in silence. Take in the different colors in the sky and appreciate the beauty of the event unfolding before your eyes. Here are a few ways you can introduce meditation into your life (Owens, n.d.):

- progressive muscle relaxation, which forces you to focus on relaxing parts of your body where you are holding tension
- body scan emanates from the Feldenkrais Method® and makes you scan your entire body to find out how you feel so you can work toward relaxation
- breath focus allows you to focus on deep breathing in order to quiet the mind; inhale positive thoughts through your nose and exhale any tension you may have through your mouth while paying attention to any physical changes that happen because of your breathing
- imagining one of your favorite places, through a practice called guided imagery, can calm your nervous system and engage your senses

There are many resources online providing guided meditations. If you don't know where to start, I recommend starting with a YouTube search for guided meditation or browsing the Calm channel. Being guided by another voice can also lead you to a state of relaxation. Practicing mindful eating is another way to incorporate meditation into your life. Say a prayer before meals or show gratitude for the meal and thank the person who prepared it. Do not eat or drink right away; engage all your senses and take notice of the smells, textures, and temperature of the food. When you are tasting the food, focus on the different flavors in your mouth without being distracted by anything else. Using these various methods of meditation can be a part of your daily life and help to keep your stress levels down.

HOW TO JOURNAL FOR STRESS RELIEF

Journaling is when you write down your thoughts and emotions in a journal. Use this as a tool to reduce stress and cope with everyday life. Keeping a journal and writing in it daily can help you cope with mental health issues, such as anxiety and depression. The benefits of journaling include the following (Benton, 2022):

- your stress triggers become more recognizable
- you can identify underlying fears that cause you to feel anxious
- it's an opportunity to practice positive self-talk that will lead to higher confidence
- you can better manage future stressful situations
- you can recognize and minimize harmful thoughts and behavior patterns

Using a journal for stress management can make you feel in control of the situations that happened to you, as well as your emotions. Sometimes life can be overwhelming and using a journal to sort through your thoughts and feelings can give your life direction and help you make positive decisions for yourself.

Steps to Start a Stress Relief Journal

It is better to start simple, with a pen and notebook. There are so many journals, including gratitude journals, music journals, and picture journals. Whatever you feel a spark of creativity for, there is the journal you can choose. It is important to establish a routine with your journaling so that it becomes a habit. Set a specific time every day in order to write in your journal for 5 to 10 minutes. The journal can be a plain notepad, or you can splurge and buy a fancy one. The choice is yours.

You can choose to have a format in how you journal. Before talking about your emotions and events of the previous day, list things you are grateful for. Whichever format you choose to use should be one that is comfortable for you to journal. Your journal could be private and personal, where you don't share its contents with anyone, or you could occasionally share with your loved ones to help you talk through your feelings. It may even be beneficial to bring your journal to therapy sessions so that you can dissect your thoughts and feelings with your mental health specialist. There is a positive effect on your life if you keep a journal.

Gratitude Journaling

Developing gratitude can stabilize your emotional well-being and reduce stress. 'Maintaining a gratitude journal makes it easy to get in the habit of focusing on the positive in your life while also reaping the benefits of journaling' (Scott, n.d.). Although you may plan to express your gratitude in your journal, remember to always show it in real life to those you appreciate. If you are grateful for your family, let them know how you feel as well as write it in your journal. Choose three things that you are grateful for and write about them in detail. Remember that at some point you will re-read what you have written, therefore it should serve as a motivation for times when you feel stressed or anxious. Do not stick to the obvious things to be grateful for. Be creative. You can express how grateful you are that you got to enjoy your favorite cake from your baker, who only uses local organic ingredients. Be grateful for the small things in your life.

EMBRACING YOUR HYGGE

Hygge (pronounced HOO-GUH) is the Danish method of happiness popularized by Meik Wiking in his book *"The Little Book of Hygge: Danish Secrets to Happy Living"*. Research shows Danish are one of the happiest communities in the world and thus, we can learn a few things from them to reduce stress. Hygge involves being in the present moment, which can enhance calmness, clarity of thought, and reduce negative behaviors and feelings. This can also calm the fight-or-flight response and create feelings of safety and peace. Anxiety is about not feeling safe and feeling out of control; Hygge encourages self-care and security and reduces your anxiety.

Hygge practice encourages a sense of community because one of its key elements is gaining social support from those around you. When you interact with your loved ones, you may become more motivated and less stressed. Hearing encouraging words will reduce negative self-talk and feelings of depression. There are various ways you can embrace your Hygge, such as (Van Syckel 2019).

- create a space where you can experience Hygge activities
- give yourself 10 extra minutes in bed
- give yourself regular breaks when you feel overwhelmed or busy
- spend some time with no electronics, TV, laptop, or phone
- spend time with your loved ones where you are fully present in the activity that you are doing, such as a hike, a hot meal, or a delightful conversation
- read a book that you enjoy or that helps you develop a new interest
- create a playlist that helps you practice Hygge; choose the music that makes you feel happy or calm as it will relax you when you feeling stressed
- bake some sweets to enjoy the dopamine rush that comes with eating sweet things
- enjoy some time playing whether it's a board game, a sport, with your children or grandchildren
- have a self-care weekend dedicated to activities that make you feel more relaxed (movie marathon, spa day, alone time)

By embracing your Hygge, you can reduce your stress and get yourself back to a happy place. The Danes may hold the secret to a happier life. You can try their ways and see what effect it has on your life, stress levels, and emotional well-being.

UNUSUAL STRESS BUSTERS TO TRY

If stress brings you down and the methods you have been using are not working, perhaps it's time to step out of your comfort zone and try something new. Buy an adult coloring book and experiment with felt pens, coloring pencils, or wax crayons so that you can color for 10 minutes or more when you feel bombarded with stress. Coloring Mandalas (a spiritual symbol in Asian cultures that represents the universal thought) helps develop creativity and is a proven method to release stress and anxiety.

When you feel stressed, try taking off your shoes and wiggle your toes; flex and relax your feet and pay attention to the movements. The simple action can relieve internal tension and wearing bright colorful socks can provide an unexpected mood uplift.

Create a happy bank of pictures and memories to uplift yourself when you are feeling low. This bank could include pictures of your loved ones, funny videos of cute animals or your favorite jokes, or anything that will put a smile on your face. Playing a prank on a loved one could also provide some needed laughter and a release of tension. Rearrange your living room or bedroom so that it feels like a new room. Watch a comedy, like a sitcom, or a romcom because humor is one of the proven methods to relieve stress and improve your emotional health.

Had I had all these tools to relieve stress during the most difficult time in my life, perhaps I would have never developed leaky gut syndrome. By using some of them, I brought my stress levels down. When I watch TV, most of the time it's a comedy. I started taking Japanese style painting classes, and learned Yoga Nidra meditation, which is an ancient method that combines guided imagery, visualization, and relaxation. I love spending time in art galleries and getting together with friends for a cup of coffee or a nature walk.

It took a very long time for me to link my overall health with the status of my gut health, even though the more stressed I would get, the worse my gut issues became. After many months of deep self-introspection and research, I started to meditate, exercise more, practice intermittent fasting, and eat a probiotic-rich diet. Day after day, my stress was getting under control and it stabilized my gut and gave my overall health an enormous boost. My menopause symptoms were easier to handle, and I just felt good. Even my autoimmune symptoms and relapses became more tamed and less frequent. It took me a long time to get here, but I'm happy I did. Where I am today, physically and emotionally, is where I hope you will be by the end of this book, too.

CONCLUSION

At the worst possible time in my life, I entered menopause as I was struggling to come to terms with my autoimmune disease. A big part of my identity was being a mother, and my son was about to leave the home and assert his independence. When I received the diagnosis of leaky gut syndrome while I was dealing with menopause symptoms, I thought my body turned against me. Struggling with weight issues had affected my self-esteem and self-image, like most women. And now, more problems. My health felt as if it was falling to pieces. I had to think about how I could feel powerful again. I knew menopause signified the beginning of a new stage in my life. Was it my chance to become a new woman?

Just like you, my symptoms used to keep me up at night; it felt easier to deny they were happening rather than face and deal with them. Recent biological changes may have caused you frustration that makes it difficult for you to enjoy time with loved ones, hobbies that you are passionate about, or even everyday activities that used to be so easy to do. I know you may dislike the person you see in the mirror. This is not your fault. You want to enjoy your life without the pain, stress, and discomfort that comes with menopause. It is possible to cope with menopause, lose weight, reduce the effects of stress, and take pleasure in your life again. *"7 Healthy Gut Habits for Women Over 40"* is the missing link you have been searching for to get the life back you once enjoyed.

This book allows you to understand the things that are happening in your body during menopause and why these symptoms are occurring. Having information about the processes that are happening in your body will reduce fear and anxiety created by ignorance. I have revealed how important your gut health is and how it fits into your overall health. The power of intermittent fasting gave me the power to control my weight. I have taught you how to use intermittent fasting as an effective tool to lose weight, maintain your hormonal balance, and support your gut health, to name a few. To support gut health, you need to eat the right foods, rich in prebiotics and probiotics, to maintain good bacteria present in the gut. This book has guided you on what diet looks like.

I didn't know the way I ate influenced my gut, thus I dedicated an entire chapter to teach you to eat mindfully and slowly to protect your gut. Knowing what to avoid to maintain gut health is also as important as knowing what to eat to promote it. I have outlined the various foods, cosmetics, and household products to avoid because of their gut-harming properties. Adopting a healthy lifestyle that includes exercise will improve your gut health, so *"7 Healthy Gut Habits for Women Over 40"* includes a chapter dedicated to exercises that support good gut health. Sleep and activities that reduce stress are also crucial for a well-functioning gut. The last chapters of the book include tips for a good night's rest and stress relief to round out the habits you need to maintain your gut health.

My story had only started after I took control of my menopause symptoms, my autoimmune disease, and leaky gut syndrome. When I started applying the tips I revealed to you, my health improved, I lost weight and regained confidence I lacked for many years. With my symptoms under control, I had more energy and motivation to live life on my own terms. I felt energetic again, and anything was possible for me. The idea of being self-employed, break free from my corporate job and start following my passions in art and design had always been on the back of my mind. I didn't think I could succeed, so I was afraid to bring it to life. Developing the habits I outlined in the book gave me enough confidence and a desire to do it. With my husband's support, I looked at our lifestyle in a busy city and long hours of commute to work. I knew it wasn't the life we wanted for our midlife. Six months later, we were living on the other side of the country close to the ocean, where I started a home staging and decorating business. It was a whole new life for me. I still enjoy keeping my healthy gut habits strong.

A lot of my family and friends have enjoyed the tips that I have revealed to you, and they are now living new lives. Heather, 47, my former co-worker, has lost weight and fell in love with yoga. She received her yoga instructor certification and opened up a gym for elderly women. By developing the habits I outlined in this book, Heather ended up gaining enough determination to begin a whole new life. We shared the enthusiasm to begin fresh because we knew we could do it. We love how we look and how we feel. Our attitude to menopause has done a complete 180°.

I know perimenopause and menopause have brought you a lot of discomfort and frustration; it is now time to bid farewell to the negativity surrounding your health. You are in control of your life. The gut influences the functions of all organs in your body, and taking care of it is the key to optimal health. The time to prioritize your gut health begins now. After you read and implement *"7 Healthy Gut Habits for Women Over 40"*, the miracle-like effects a healthy and happy gut can bring into your life will surprise you!

WOULD YOU LEAVE A REVIEW?

Thank you for purchasing my book and taking the time to read it. If *"7 Healthy Gut Habits for Women Over 40"* has had a positive impact on your life, please leave a review on Amazon. My intention was to deliver to you seven methods to heal your gut with intermittent fasting, exercise, and other self-care methods; if I achieved my mandate, I would love to hear all about your experience. I would love to hear how you applied these habits to your life, how much weight you have lost, and how you feel about yourself now. A review can also serve as a lighthouse for women who may seek direction in the sea of perimenopause and menopause symptoms; your review can help them turn their life around too.

I hope this book will help you cultivate the attitude you need to overcome your perimenopause and menopause symptoms. Good health is not a singular road that leads to one destination; rather, good health is a busy highway that has many twists and turns. It is multi-faceted and complex. Understanding the different factors that affect your gut health can drive you toward a fulfilling life that is supported by good health. After all, you are just as healthy as your gut.

Scan the QR code below to leave a review!

PLEASE LEAVE ME A REVIEW TO BENEFIT OTHERS JUST LIKE YOU!

YOUR GIFT

7 HEALTHY GUT HABITS FOR WOMEN OVER 40 WORKBOOK

Congratulations, you did it; you finished the book! And now, the fun part — forming your new habits. Once you form them, you'll be well on your way to a healthier, more fulfilling life, to a lifestyle you love, and to making your 40s and beyond your best years. However, it's often difficult to make consistent positive changes and stick to new habits.

I created this workbook to help you succeed. If you haven't downloaded it earlier, now is the time.

You can track your habits in multiple ways. It's important to be conscious of your thoughts and committed to your new habits. Record your intentions, plans, thoughts, and results in the workbook. Take small steps. Strive for progress, not perfection. Forgive yourself when you skip a day. Commit to the next action. Reward yourself for every checkmark on your list. Give your best to form the habits, and before you know it, your new habits will give you your life back.

Get immediate access to the bonus by following this link https://larawestbooks.com/workbook or scanning this QR Code:

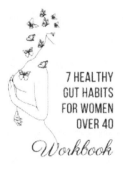

ALSO BY LARA WEST

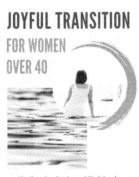

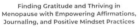

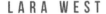

https://books2read.com/joyfultransition

Within the pages of this book you'll discover the profound impact of positive mindset strategies, guiding you toward a life brimming with joy, gratitude, and the freedom to enjoy every moment. You'll be equipped with strategies to shift your perspective, allowing you to see perimenopause and menopause as a positive, life-affirming experience.

If you resonate with holistic approaches to well-being, believe in the profound connection between mind and body, and are ready to embrace your 40s and beyond with joy, this guide is your trusted friend and mentor on this transformative journey.

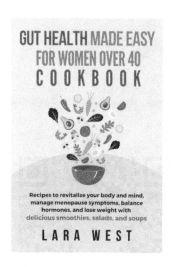

https://books2read.com/guthealthmadeeasy

This transformative cookbook unveils the secrets to conquering perimenopause and menopause symptoms through nourishing meals made with wholesome ingredients. In it, Lara simplifies the essential message: by embracing nutrient-dense superfoods and intermittent fasting, you can soothe your body, balance hormones, get mental clarity, and shed excess weight naturally.

If you're a woman over 40 looking to regain your vitality and take control of your health, "Gut Health Made Easy for Women over 40" is your essential playbook for solving menopause troubles and finding vitality in every meal And if you love comfort food with a health-conscious twist, then you'll adore this cookbook and its delicious recipes.

REFERENCES

Alcohol and the digestive system. (n.d.). Alcohol Think Again. https://alcoholthinkagain.com.au/alcohol-your-health/alcohol-and-long-term-health/alcohol-and-the-digestive-system/

Alkon, C. (2018, December 31). *Fitness needs after age 40: Exercise recommendations for perimenopause and menopause.* Everyday Health. https://www.everydayhealth.com/menopause/know-about-midlife-exercise-needs/

Alternative treatments for insomnia. (n.d.). WebMD. https://www.webmd.com/sleep-disorders/alternative-treatments-for-insomnia

Andriakos, J. (2016, March 21). *How to eliminate sugar from your diet in 21 days.* Health. https://www.health.com/nutrition/slash-sugar-challenge

Atkinson, D. (2019, May 9). *Why HIIT injury risks are high for women in menopause.* Flipping Fifty. https://www.flippingfifty.com/exercise-injury-women-in-menopause/

Becker, S. L., & Manson, J. E. (2020). *Menopause, the gut microbiome, and weight gain.* Menopause, Publish Ahead of Print. https://doi.org/10.1097/gme.0000000000001702

Benton, E. (2022, April 26). *How to use journaling for stress relief.* Psych Central. https://psychcentral.com/stress/how-to-begin-journaling-for-stress-relief#benefits-of-journaling

Berk, J. E. (2019, January 27). *5 reasons why you're eating too fast.* Jenny Eden Berk. https://www.jennyedenberk.com/blogroll/5-reasons-why-youre-eating-too-fast

Beukema, M., Faas, M. M., & de Vos, P. (2020). The effects of different dietary fiber pectin structures on the gastrointestinal immune barrier: Impact via gut microbiota and direct effects on immune cells. *Experimental & Molecular Medicine, 52*(9), 1364–1376. https://doi.org/10.1038/s12276-020-0449-2

Bjarnadottir, A. (2019, June 19). *Mindful eating 101 — A beginner's guide.* Healthline. https://www.healthline.com/nutrition/mindful-eating-guide

Bokor, V. (2020, September 24). *Intermittent fasting and hormones: For a better balance.* WeFast. https://www.wefast.care/articles/intermittent-fasting-and-hormones

Bonsall, D. A. (n.d.). *The digestive system.* Patient. https://patient.info/news-and-features/the-digestive-system

Breus, M. (2022, September 9). *How to fall asleep fast.* The Sleep Doctor. https://thesleepdoctor.com/sleep-hygiene/how-to-fall-asleep-fast/

Brighten, J. (2022, September 30). *Connection between gut health, menopause, and perimenopause.* Dr. Jolene Brighten. https://drbrighten.com/gut-health-menopause-and-perimenopause/

Carr, K. (n.d.). *A-Z Quotes.* Retrieved October 13, 2022, from https://www.azquotes.com/quote/810689?ref=digestion

Cherney, K. (2019, February 5). *Effects of menopause on the body.* Healthline. https://www.healthline.com/health/menopause/hrt-effects-on-body#

Ciccolini, K. (2018, January 30). *If your gut could talk: 10 things you should know.* Healthline. https://www.healthline.com/health/digestive-health/things-your-gut-wants-you-to-know

Clauss, M., Gérard, P., Mosca, A., & Leclerc, M. (2021). Interplay Between Exercise and Gut Microbiome in the Context of Human Health and Performance. *Frontiers in Nutrition,* 8. https://doi.org/10.3389/fnut.2021.637010

Cleveland Clinic. (2021, October 5). *Menopause: Age, stages, signs, symptoms & treatment.* Cleveland Clinic. https://my.clevelandclinic.org/health/diseases/21841-menopause

Cleveland Clinic. (2022, March 14). *What are prebiotics and what do they do?* Cleveland Clinic. https://health.clevelandclinic.org/what-are-prebiotics/

Collins, J. (2020, September 14). *What are prebiotics?* WebMD. https://www.webmd.com/digestive-disorders/prebiotics-overview

Coyle, D. (2017). *8 surprising things that harm your gut bacteria.* Healthline. https://www.healthline.com/nutrition/8-things-that-harm-gut-bacteria

Darmody, J. (2018, May 8). *6 unusual stress busters for when you're feeling over-whelmed.* Silicon Republic. https://www.siliconrepublic.com/advice/stress-busters-tips

Davis, J. L. (n.d.). *Tips to reduce stress in women over 50.* WebMD. Retrieved October 21, 2022, from https://www.webmd.com/women/guide/women-over-50-tips-to-reduce-stress

Dix, M., & Klein, E. (2018, July 2). *Understanding gut health: Signs of an unhealthy gut and what to do about it.* Healthline. https://www.healthline.com/health/gut-health

Dorr, B. (2022, September 14). *Contributor: In the misdiagnosis of menopause, what needs to change?* AJMC. https://www.ajmc.com/view/contributor-in-the-misdiagnosis-of-menopause-what-needs-to-change-

Eske, J. (2019, August 21). *What to know about leaky gut syndrome.* Medical News Today. https://www.medicalnewstoday.com/articles/326117

Felson, S. (2017, January 26). *What are probiotics?* WebMD. https://www.webmd.com/digestive-disorders/what-are-probiotics

GIS. (2007, July). *Stress and your gut.* Gastrointestinal Society. https://badgut.org/information-centre/a-z-digestive-topics/stress-and-your-gut/

Gordon, D. (2021, July 13). *73% of women don't treat their menopause symptoms, new survey shows.* Forbes. https://www.forbes.com/sites/debgordon/2021/07/13/73-of-women-dont-treat-their-menopause-symptoms-new-survey-shows/?sh=77a4634b454f

Gunnars, K. (2018, November 13). *Probiotics 101: A simple beginner's guide.* Healthline. https://www.healthline.com/nutrition/probiotics-101

Gunnars, K. (2020, April 20). *Intermittent fasting 101 — the ultimate beginner's guide.* Healthline. https://www.healthline.com/nutrition/intermittent-fasting-guide

Hannan, Md. A., Rahman, Md. A., Rahman, M. S., Sohag, A. A. M., Dash, R., Hossain, K. S., Farjana, M., & Uddin, M. J. (2020). Intermittent fasting, a possible priming tool for host defense against SARS-CoV-2 infection: Crosstalk among calorie restriction, autophagy and immune response. *Immunology Letters, 226,* 38–45. https://doi.org/10.1016/j.imlet.2020.07.001

Healthline Medical Network. (2018, October 26). *What Does Gamma Aminobutyric Acid (GABA) Do?* Healthline. https://www.healthline.com/health/gamma-aminobutyric-acid#

Henry Ford Health Staff. (2021, February 24). *How lack of sleep can affect gut health.* Henry Ford. https://www.henryford.com/blog/2021/02/sleep-affects-gut-health

Hester, L., Dang, D., Barker, C. J., Heath, M., Mesiya, S., Tienabeso, T., & Watson, K. (2021). Evening wear of blue-blocking glasses for sleep and mood disorders: A systematic review. *Chronobiology International, 38*(10), 1375–1383. https://doi.org/10.1080/07420528.2021.1930029

Hewings-Martin, Y. (2017, September 15). *Why chocolate is good for your gut.* Medical News Today. https://www.medicalnewstoday.com/articles/319408

Hippocrates quotes about health, food and medicine >. (2020, August 8).

Wise Owl Quotes. https://wiseowlquotes.com/hippocrates/

Househam, A. M., Peterson, C. T., Mills, P. J., & Chopra, D. (2017). The effects of stress and meditation on the immune system, human microbiota, and epigenetics. *Advances in Mind-Body Medicine*, 31(4), 10–25. https://pubmed. ncbi.nlm.nih.gov/29306937/

How meditation heals the gut-brain axis, no probiotics. (n.d.). EOC Institute. https://eocinstitute.org/meditation/beyond-probiotics-how-meditation-heals-the-gut-brain-axis-stress/

Huizen, J. (2020, December 24). *How gut microbes contribute to good sleep.* Medical News Today. https://www.medicalnewstoday.com/articles/how-gut-microbes-contribute-to-good-sleep#The-microbiota-gut-brain-axis

Huizen, J. (2022, September 16). *Abdominal or stomach pain at night: Common causes and prevention.* Medical News Today. https://www.medicalnewsto day.com/articles/317690#

Humphreys, C. (2020). Intestinal permeability. *Textbook of Natural Medicine*, 166-177.e4. https://doi.org/10.1016/b978-0-323-43044-9.00019-4

Insomnia. (2017, October 18). NHS. https://www.nhs.uk/conditions/ insomnia/

Izquierdo, A. (2021, November 2). *Can You Take Too Many Probiotics?* Omnibiotic Life. https://www.omnibioticlife.com/can-you-take-too-many-probiotics/

John Hopkins Medicine. (2019). *Anatomy of the endocrine system.* Johns Hopkins Medicine. https://www.hopkinsmedicine.org/health/wellness-and-prevention/anatomy-of-the-endocrine-system

Kandola, A. (2019, April 2). *5 reasons why sugar is bad for you.* Medical News Today. https://www.medicalnewstoday.com/articles/324854

Kazan, J. (2021, October 4). *What women over 50 need to know before taking probiotics.* Yahoo. https://www.yahoo.com/lifestyle/women-over-50-know-taking-060000368.html

Kozmor, T. (n.d.). *3 ways exercise affects the gut.* Ixcela. https://ixcela.com/ resources/3-ways-exercise-affects-the-gut.html

Laurence, E. (2021, March 26). *I'm a gastroenterologist, and this is what happens when you cut added sugar.* Well+Good. https://www.wellandgood.com/ cutting-sugar-affects-gut-health/

Leaky gut syndrome. (n.d.). Cleveland Clinic. https://my.clevelandclinic.org/ health/diseases/22724-leaky-gut-syndrome

Leonard, J. (2020, April 16). *Seven ways to do intermittent fasting.* Medical News

Today. https://www.medicalnewstoday.com/articles/322293#tips-for-maintaining-intermittent-fasting

Lee, K. (n.d.). *Guide to prebiotic fiber and importance of gut health.* ROWDY. https://rowdybars.com/blogs/rowdy-blog/what-is-prebiotic-fiber

Lindberg, S. (2020, September 1). *How to exercise safely during intermittent fasting.* Healthline. https://www.healthline.com/health/how-to-exercise-safely-intermittent-fasting

LoveBug Probiotics. (n.d.). *13 foods that are terrible for your gut health.* LoveBug Probiotics. https://lovebugprobiotics.com/blogs/news/13-foods-that-are-terrible-for-your-gut-health

MacGill, M. (2018, June 26). *Gut microbiota: Definition, importance, and medical uses.* Medical News Today. https://www.medicalnewstoday.com/articles/307998

MedicineNet. (n.d.). *How long do you need to fast for autophagy?* MedicineNet. https://www.medicinenet.com/how_long_do_you_need_to_fast_for_autophagy/article.htm

Menopause and weight gain. (n.d.). Better Health. https://www.betterhealth.vic.gov.au/health/conditionsandtreatments/menopause-and-weight-gain

Monda, V., Villano, I., Messina, A., Valenzano, A., Esposito, T., Moscatelli, F., Viggiano, A., Cibelli, G., Chieffi, S., Monda, M., & Messina, G. (2017). Exercise modifies the gut microbiota with positive health effects. *Oxidative Medicine and Cellular Longevity,* 2017, 1–8. https://doi.org/10.1155/2017/3831972

Nair, P. M. K., & Khawale, P. G. (2016). Role of therapeutic fasting in women's health: An overview. *Journal of Mid-Life Health,* 7(2), 61. https://doi.org/10.4103/0976-7800.185325

Nathoo, S. (2022, March 15). *Digestive problems? Menopause might be to blame.* Orlando Health. https://www.orlandohealth.com/content-hub/digestive-problems-menopause-might-be-to-blame

National Center for Complementary and Integrative Health. (2021, January). *Melatonin: What you need to know.* NCCIH. https://www.nccih.nih.gov/health/melatonin-what-you-need-to-know

Nilsen, A. (2002, November). *Ultimate spaghetti carbonara recipe.* BBC Good Food. https://www.bbcgoodfood.com/recipes/ultimate-spaghetti-carbonara-recipe

Northwestern Medicine. (n.d.). *7 reasons to listen to your gut.* Northwestern

Medicine. https://www.nm.org/healthbeat/healthy-tips/7-reasons-to-listen-to-your-gut

Nunez, K., & Lamoreux, K. (2020, July 20). *Why do we sleep?* Healthline. https://www.healthline.com/health/why-do-we-sleep#

Owens, B. (n.d.). *Meditation + gut health: How are they related?* Conscious Movements. https://www.consciousmovements.com/body-mind-blog/meditation-gut-health

Palsdottir, H. (2019, June 14). *Does eating fast make you gain more weight?* Healthline; Healthline Media. https://www.healthline.com/nutrition/eating-fast-causes-weight-gain

Palsdottir, H. (2022, January 5). *11 probiotic foods that are super healthy.* Healthline. https://www.healthline.com/nutrition/11-super-healthy-probiotic-foods

Payne, J. M. (2021, February 18). *Why you should exercise your way through menopause.* Lancaster General Health. https://www.lancastergeneralhealth.org/health-hub-home/2021/february/why-you-should-exercise-your-way-through-menopause

Pelz, M. (2020, October 6). *How fasting can help you balance your hormones (estrogen) - part 2.* YouTube. https://www.youtube.com/watch?app=desktop&v=P0yApcHn_gA

Pietrangelo, A. (2017, May 4). *Menopause and pregnancy: What you should know.* Healthline. https://www.healthline.com/health/menopause/menopause-pregnancy#

Prados, A. (2022, January 19). *Is water the forgotten nutrient for your gut microbiota?* Gut Microbiota for Health. https://www.gutmicrobiotaforhealth.com/is-water-the-forgotten-nutrient-for-your-gut-microbiota/

Pratt, E. (2018, January 12). *Research Says Exercise Also Improves Your Gut Bacteria.* Healthline. https://www.healthline.com/health-news/exercise-improves-your-gut-bacteria

Raman, R. (2021, May 19). *What are postbiotics? A comprehensive overview.* Healthline. https://www.healthline.com/nutrition/postbiotics

Rowles, A., & Shoemaker, S. (2017, May 22). *14 simple ways to stop eating lots of sugar.* Healthline; Healthline Media. https://www.healthline.com/nutrition/14-ways-to-eat-less-sugar

Ruscio, M. (2020, July 4). *Probiotics for leaky gut.* Dr. Ruscio. https://drruscio.com/probiotics-for-leaky-gut/

Santos, A. (2021, July 1). *Why you can't seem to stay asleep (plus, how to finally catch some zzz's).* Healthline. https://www.healthline.com/health/healthy-sleep/why-cant-i-stay-asleep

Scott, E. (n.d.). *How to maintain a gratitude journal for stress relief.* Verywell Mind. https://www.verywellmind.com/writing-in-a-gratitude-journal-for-stress-relief-3144887

Scottish Government. (2022, October 17). *Menopause and your mental wellbeing.* NHS Inform. https://www.nhsinform.scot/healthy-living/womens-health/later-years-around-50-years-and-over/menopause-and-post-menopause-health/menopause-and-your-mental-wellbeing

Seladi-Schulman, J. (2019, December 4). *What is SIFO and how can it affect your gut health?* Healthline. https://www.healthline.com/health/sifo

Semeco, A. (2016, June 8). *The 19 best prebiotic foods you should eat.* Healthline. https://www.healthline.com/nutrition/19-best-prebiotic-foods

SIBO (small intestinal bacterial overgrowth). (n.d.). Cleveland Clinic. https://my.clevelandclinic.org/health/diseases/21820-small-intestinal-bacterial-overgrowth-sibo

Silva, A. L. (2020, March 3). *Intermittent fasting: For your gut's sake.* Gutxy. https://www.gutxy.com/blog/intermittent-fasting-for-your-guts-sake/

Slumber Yard Team. (2021, June 1). *The gut-sleep connection: How to heal your gut for better sleep.* My Slumber Yard. https://myslumberyard.com/blog/the-gut-sleep-connection/

Spencer, C. (2021, July 4). Loss of confidence and self-esteem. My Menopause Centre. https://www.mymenopausecentre.com/symptoms/loss-of-confidence-and-self-esteem/

Sperlazza, C. (2021, April 15). *What is metabolic flexibility and how can you achieve it?* Bulletproof. https://www.bulletproof.com/diet/weight-loss/metabolic-flexibility/

Spritzler, F. (2019, June 18). *Does eating slowly help you lose weight?* Healthline. https://www.healthline.com/nutrition/eating-slowly-and-weight-loss#

Spritzler, F. (2020, April 27). *What to know about inulin, a healthful prebiotic.* Medical News Today. https://www.medicalnewstoday.com/articles/318593

St. Pierre, B. (2018, February 6). *All about eating slowly.* Precision Nutrition; Precision Nutrition. https://www.precisionnutrition.com/all-about-slow-eating

Staub, D. (n.d.). *What you need to know about prebiotics.* Columbia University

Department of Surgery. https://columbiasurgery.org/news/2017/02/09/what-you-need-know-about-prebiotics

Stuart, A. (n.d.). *Menopause, weight gain, and exercise tips*. WebMD. https://www.webmd.com/menopause/guide/menopause-weight-gain-and-exercise-tips

Sweet, W. (2022a, April 27). *Sleep all night: The connection between menopause & sleepless nights*. My Menopause Transformation. https://www.mymenopausetransformation.com/sleepless-nights/the-connection-between-menopause-and-your-sleepless-nights/

Sweet, W. (2022b, July 19). *The water you drink & why it affects gut health in midlife*. My Menopause Transformation. https://www.mymenopausetransformation.com/menopause-gut-health/new-research-the-water-you-drink-and-why-it-affects-gut-health-in-midlife/

The Healthline Editorial Team. (2014, August 18). *Healthy cosmetics*. Healthline. https://www.healthline.com/health/beauty-skin-care-cosmetics

The Surprising Link Between Sleep and Digestion. (2022, March 11). Reverie. https://www.reverie.com/blog/sleep-and-digestion.html

25 weird breaks for stress relief. (2014, June 18). KU Faculty and Staff Wellness. https://wellness.ku.edu/25-weird-breaks-stress-relief

Van Oord, G. (2019, May 8). *The gut-brain axis explained in plain English*. Diet vs Disease. https://www.dietvsdisease.org/gut-brain-axis/

Van Sickel, E. (2019, January 3). *Eight hygge ideas for your mental health*. Restored Hope Counseling Services. https://www.restoredhopecounselingservices.com/blog/2019/1/2/eight-hygge-ideas-for-your-mental-health

Vandergriendt, C. (2020, July 16). *What's the difference between dopamine and serotonin?* Healthline. https://www.healthline.com/health/dopamine-vs-serotonin#

Vanner, C. (2020, December 22). *Intermittent fasting diet: Tips for success*. Forkly. https://www.forkly.com/food-trends/intermittent-fasting-diet-10-tips-for-success/

Vazquez, S. M. (2020, August 12). *The best probiotics for women over 50 for a healthy gut*. Woman's World. https://www.womansworld.com/gallery/health/best-probiotic-women-over-50-156818

Veloso, H. (n.d.). *FODMAP diet: What you need to know*. Hopkins Medicine. https://www.hopkinsmedicine.org/health/wellness-and-prevention/

fodmap-diet-what-you-need-to-know

Vivekanandarajah, S. (n.d.). *How too much sugar affects the gut microbiome*. Dr. Suhirdan Vivekanandarajah. https://sydneygastroenterologist.com.au/blog/how-too-much-sugar-affects-the-gut-microbiome/

WebMD. (2014, September 8). *Ketosis*. WebMD. https://www.webmd.com/diabetes/type-1-diabetes-guide/what-is-ketosis#1

WebMD. (2017). *Working out when you're over 50*. WebMD. https://www.webmd.com/fitness-exercise/ss/slideshow-exercise-after-age-50

WebMD Editorial Contributors. (n.d.-a). *Menopause*. WebMD. https://www.webmd.com/menopause/guide/menopause-basics#091e9c5e800078f3-3-12

WebMD Editorial Contributors. (n.d.-b). *Sleepless nights plague many women in middle age*. WebMD. https://www.webmd.com/sleep-disorders/news/20170907/sleepless-nights-plague-many-women-in-middle-age

WebMD Editorial Contributors. (n.d.-c). *What to know about intermittent fasting for women after 50*. WebMD. https://www.webmd.com/healthy-aging/what-to-know-about-intermittent-fasting-for-women-after-50

WebMD Editorial Contributors. (n.d.-d). *What to know about resistant starches*. WebMD. https://www.webmd.com/diet/what-to-know-resistant-starches

What's the difference between probiotics and prebiotics? (n.d.). SCL Health. https://www.sclhealth.org/blog/2019/07/difference-between-probiotics-and-prebiotics/

Whittel, N. (2022, August 6). *Autophagy: The fountain of youth for your cells*. Naomi Whittel. https://naomiw.com/blogs/health/autophagy

Why chewing food and eating slowly improves your health. (2021, April 2). Nathan Mogren DMD. https://mogrendental.com/why-chewing-food-and-eating-slowly-improves-your-health/

Wolkin, J. (2015, August 27). *Mindful eating for a healthier brain-gut connection*. Mindful. https://www.mindful.org/mindful-eating-for-a-healthier-brain-gut-connection/

Women's Voices for the Earth. (n.d.). *Health hazards in scented cleaning products*. Women's Voices for the Earth. https://womensvoices.org/beyondthelabel/health-hazards-in-scented-cleaning-products/

Woods, B. (2021, March 9). *When is the best time to take prebiotics?* Omnibiotic Life. https://www.omnibioticlife.com/when-to-take-prebiotics/

Yeager, S. (2022, April 11). *Why menopausal women should do HIIT workouts*. Feisty Menopause. https://www.feistymenopause.com/blog/the-best-hiit-workouts-for-menopausal-women

Zelman, K. M. (2005, January 5). *Slow down, you eat too fast.* WebMD; WebMD. https://www.webmd.com/diet/obesity/features/slow-down-you-eat-too-fast

Made in the USA
Las Vegas, NV
18 April 2024

88873619R00095